CONTINUOUS MEASUREMENT OF BLOOD OXYGEN SATURATION IN THE HIGH RISK PATIENT

Theory and Practice in Monitoring Mixed Venous Oxygen Saturation

Volume 2

Edited by Patrick J. Fahey, M.D.

This publication was sponsored under an educational grant from
Oximetrix, Inc.

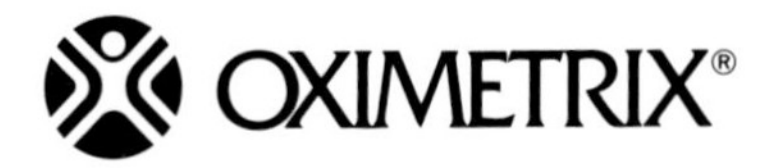

Beach International, Inc.
P.O. Box 28364
11858 Bernardo Plaza Court
San Diego, California 92128

Distributed by
Oximetrix, Inc.
1212 Terra Bella Avenue
Mountain View, California 94043

Library of Congress Catalog
Number 84-073528

International Standard Book
Number 0-942210-21-2

Printed in the United States
of America

PREFACE

Mixed venous oxygen saturation ($S\bar{v}O_2$) reflects the balance between oxygen supply and overall tissue oxygen demand. Changes in $S\bar{v}O_2$ values reflect changes in oxygen demand or cardiorespiratory function that threaten the adequacy of oxygen delivery or the tissue's ability to metabolize oxygen.

A patient may be anemic secondary to hemodilution, hypoxemic because of pulmonary edema, poorly perfused because of left ventricular failure, or unable to compensate for increases in oxygen demand. In all of these situations, continuous measurement of $S\bar{v}O_2$ serves as an early warning and can alert the clinician to the need for therapeutic intervention that prevents more serious crises from occurring.

This monograph provides the most recent research and thinking on continuous measurement of $S\bar{v}O_2$ and its use in assessment and management of the high-risk patient. It is a compilation of papers presented in a seminar entitled "The Value of Continuous Monitoring of Mixed Venous Oxygen Saturation" held in conjunction with the 49th Annual Scientific Assembly of the American College of Chest

Physicians. Chapter 1 of the monograph is reprinted from Volume 1 of the series and reviews the fundamentals of oxygen transport physiology in the context of hemodynamic monitoring. All of the other chapters are new material. Chapter 6 supplies background on the theory and development of the OXIMETRIX® Opticath® Oximetry System. This material was not a part of the ACCP Seminar.

Patrick J. Fahey, M.D.
Associate Professor of Medicine
Pulmonary Division
Loyola University of Chicago
Maywood, Illinois

PRESENTERS

Arnold Aberman, M.D., F.A.C.P.
Professor of Medicine
University of Toronto
Physician-in-Chief
Mount Sinai Hospital
Toronto, Ontario, Canada

Patrick J. Fahey, M.D.
Associate Professor of Medicine
Director, Medical Intensive Care Unit
Pulmonary Division
Foster G. McGaw Hospital
Loyola University of Chicago
Maywood, Illinois

Joel M. Gore, M.D.
Assistant Professor of Medicine
Clinical Director of CCU
University of Massachusetts Medical School
Worcester, Massachusetts

John C. McMichan, M.B., B.S., Ph.D.,
Consultant in Intensive Care and Anesthesiology
Mayo Clinic
Assistant Professor of Anesthesiology
Mayo Medical School
Director, Surgical and Trauma Intensive Care Unit
St. Mary's Hospital
Rochester, Minnesota

Paul M. Stevens, M.D.
Professor of Medicine
Baylor College of Medicine
Director of Medical Intensive Care
Methodist Hospital
Houston, Texas

CONTRIBUTORS

Kathi M. Senelly, B.S.
Clinical Engineer
Oximetrix, Inc.
Mountain View, California

John M. Sperinde, Ph.D.
Vice President
Clinical Engineering
Oximetrix, Inc.
Mountain View, California

CONTINUING EDUCATION INFORMATION

PROFESSIONAL CREDIT

A passing score of 75% is required to obtain professional credit. Self-paced learning programs are appropriate to submit as Category E for CCRN recertification.

The University of California, San Diego School of Medicine designates this continuing medical education activity for three (3) credit hours in Category 1 of the Physician's Recognition Award of the American Medical Association and for the Certification Program of the California Medical Association.

This offering for three (3) contact hours is sponsored by The Self-Paced Continuing Education Program, Health Education International, Inc., which has been granted approval of its total program of continuing education in nursing by the Western Regional Accrediting Committee of the American Nurses' Association.

Provider is approved by the California Board of Registered Nursing, Provider Number 04960, for three (3) contact hours.

CONTINUING EDUCATION INSTRUCTIONS

The pretest and posttest that accompany this book are designed to increase your understanding of the content according to the educational objectives listed below. Read the objectives and test your baseline knowledge by answering the questions in the pretest. (Answers to the pretest can be found on page 90.)

After reading the book, complete the posttest found on page 93. If you wish to obtain continuing education credit for completing this learning program, see the enrollment announcement on page 99 or contact Health Education International, Inc., P.O. Box 28364, San Diego, CA 92128, (619) 451-0342.

LEARNING OBJECTIVES

Based on the content of this monograph, the reader should be able to:

1. Describe the principles and components of oximetry systems.
2. Explain the principles of normal oxygen physiology.
3. Discuss the clinical usefulness of the OXIMETRIX® Opticath® Oximetry System for the cardiac patient.
4. Appraise the clinical usefulness of continuous $S\bar{v}O_2$ monitoring in the patient with respiratory failure.
5. Analyze the practical benefits of continuous $S\bar{v}O_2$ monitoring in all high-risk patients.

CONTINUOUS MEASUREMENT OF BLOOD OXYGEN SATURATION IN THE HIGH RISK PATIENT

PRETEST*

1. The method used for *in vivo* measurement of mixed venous oxygen saturation involves:
   a. Counting oxygen molecules
   b. Analyzing light reflected by the blood cells
   c. Tagging oxyhemoglobin
   d. Comparing weight difference between hemoglobin and oxyhemoglobin

2. Performance of the fiberoptic system of the OXIMETRIX® Oximetry catheter is reflected in:
   a. The intensity bars at the bottom of the strip recording
   b. The stability of the $S\bar{v}O_2$ values
   c. The sharpness of the waveforms obtained
   d. The digital display

3. On the arterial side of the oxyhemoglobin dissociation curve:
   a. Small changes in PO_2 result in large changes in saturation
   b. Oxygen saturation ranges from 60% to 70%
   c. As the PO_2 decreases from 90 mm Hg to 60 mm Hg, saturation will only decrease 5%
   d. None of the above

*Answers to the pretest can be found on page 90.
There is only one correct answer for each question.

4. During insertion of a pulmonary artery catheter, as the catheter is advanced from the right atrium to the right ventricle and pulmonary artery, oxygen saturations normally:
   a. Change very little
   b. Decrease significantly
   c. Increase significantly
   d. None of the above

5. Continuous $S\bar{v}O_2$ monitoring can be useful in:
   a. Weaning patients from intra-aortic balloon counterpulsation
   b. Determining prognosis
   c. Weaning patients from mechanical ventilation
   d. All of the above

6. According to the Fick equation, oxygen consumption is a function of cardiac output and:
   a. PaO_2
   b. $S\bar{v}O_2$
   c. $C\bar{v}O_2$
   d. $CaO_2 - CvO_2$

7. Changes in $S\bar{v}O_2$ can reflect alterations in:
   a. Arterial oxygen content
   b. Cardiac output
   c. Tissue oxygen consumption
   d. All of the above

8. Studies have shown that during endotracheal suctioning:
   a. Declines in $S\bar{v}O_2$ frequently outdistance falls in arterial oxygen levels
   b. Declines in arterial oxygen levels usually exceed declines in $S\bar{v}O_2$
   c. Arterial oxygen levels fall significantly, but $S\bar{v}O_2$ levels are not affected
   d. $S\bar{v}O_2$ and arterial oxygen levels are not significantly altered

TABLE OF CONTENTS

® Registered Trademark of Oximetrix, Inc.

FUNDAMENTALS OF OXYGEN TRANSPORT PHYSIOLOGY IN A HEMODYNAMIC MONITORING CONTEXT*

1

Arnold Aberman, M.D., F.A.C.P.**

This presentation is focused on the fundamentals of oxygen transport physiology in a hemodynamic monitoring context. The oxyhemoglobin dissociation curve will be reviewed, and blood oxygen content, oxygen transport and oxygen consumption will be discussed.***

*This chapter is reprinted from Volume 1 published in 1983, as it supplies the background information and fundamentals of oxygen transport physiology in a hemodynamic monitoring context. All other chapters are newly published material.

**Mount Sinai Hospital
600 University Avenue, Suite 427
Toronto, Ontario, Canada M5G 1X5

***See the list at the end of the chapter for definitions of acronyms.

Hemoglobin combines reversibly with oxygen to form oxyhemoglobin. The percent saturation is the amount of oxyhemoglobin over the total amount of hemoglobin, both reduced and oxygenated, as shown in Figure 1.

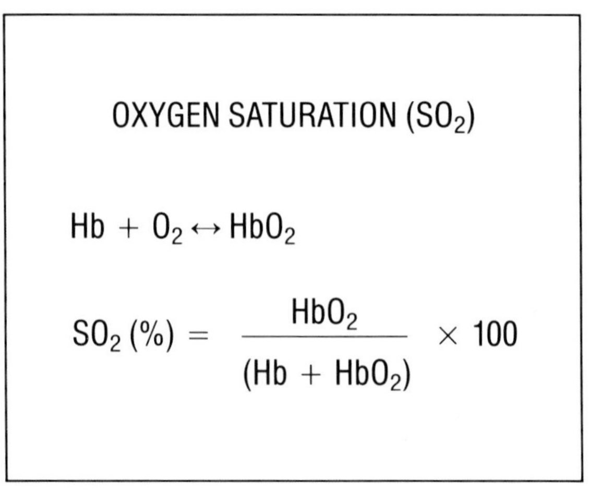

Figure 1

Saturation is related to PO_2 via the oxyhemoglobin dissociation curve illustrated in Figure 2. This curve should be familiar to most of you, but let me review some important features.

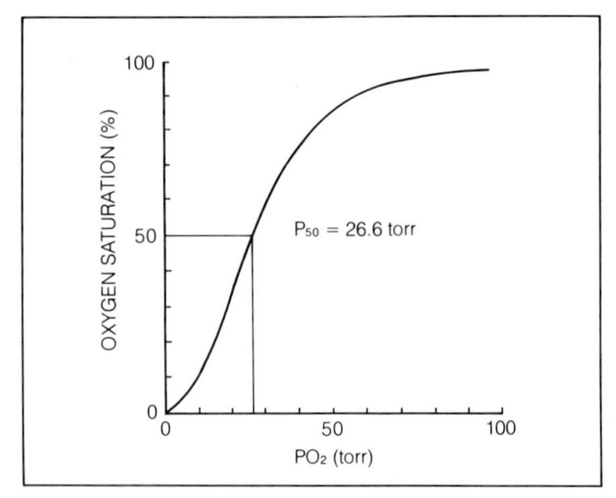

Figure 2

At a normal arterial PO_2 of 90 mm Hg the saturation is 97%. If the PO_2 decreases from 90 mm Hg to 60 mm Hg (a decrease of 33%), the saturation will only decrease from 97% to 92%—a fall of 5%. Thus, on the arterial side saturation is well protected from major changes caused by decreases in arterial PO_2.

On the venous side the picture is somewhat different. The normal venous PO_2 of approximately 40 mm Hg has a capillary saturation of 75%. Because of the steep nature of the curve on venous values, small changes in venous PO_2 get translated into large changes in venous saturation. Of course, that has important implications with respect to oxygen unloading at a tissue level.

The next term I want to define is blood oxygen content. Blood oxygen content answers the following question. In 100 ml of blood, how much oxygen is there? As you know, the oxygen exists both dissolved and combined with hemoglobin. The amount dissolved can be estimated by multiplying the PO_2 times .0031, the solubility coefficient. The amount combined with hemoglobin can be estimated by multiplying 1.38 times hemoglobin times saturation, where 1.38 is the maximum, in milliliters oxygen, that one gram of hemoglobin can combine with when fully saturated. In the literature the number ranges from 1.34 to 1.39. In the example illustrated in Figure 3, a normal person with a hemoglobin of 15 gm/dl, a PO_2 of 100 mm Hg and a saturation of 97% has 0.3 ml of oxygen dissolved per 100 ml blood. The amount combined with hemoglobin is 20.1 ml, for a total amount of oxygen of 20.4 ml of oxygen per 100 ml of blood.

BLOOD OXYGEN CONTENT (CO_2)

($ml\ O_2/100\ ml\ blood = Vol\ \%$)

O_2 Dissolved + O_2 Combined with Hemoglobin

$0.0031 \times PO_2 + 1.38 \times Hb \times SO_2$

Example:

$Hb = 15\ gm\%,\ PO_2 = 100\ mm\ Hg,\ SO_2 = 97\%$

$CO_2 = (0.0031 \times 100) + (1.38 \times 15 \times .97)$

$CO_2 = .3 + 20.1$

$CO_2 = 20.4\ Vol\ \%$

Figure 3

You will notice that the vast majority of oxygen, over 98% in this example, exists combined with hemoglobin. Only a trivial amount is dissolved—less than 2%. Therefore, if you were to ask me what role does PaO_2 play in contributing to oxygen content, I hope you would agree that directly it plays a very minimal role. It is important, of course, but its importance is that PaO_2 is a major determining factor in saturation.

You can estimate oxygen content by ignoring the amount of oxygen dissolved and considering only the amount combined with hemoglobin. Oxygen content can be estimated as simply 1.38 times hemoglobin times saturation. That will introduce only a trivial error in the calculation of content.

Finally, remember that if arterial PaO_2 falls from 100 mm Hg to 60 mm Hg, a decrease of 40% in this example, saturation only decreases by some 5%. Therefore, if the PaO_2 falls from 100 mm Hg to 60 mm Hg, content will only fall by some 6-7%, another important clinical point shown in Figure 4.

$Pa0_2$ (mm Hg)	$Sa0_2$* (%)	$Ca0_2$** (vol %)
50	85	15.4
60	91	16.4
70	94	17.0
100	97.5	17.6

*pH: 7.40, T: 37°C
**Hb: 13 gm/dl

Figure 4

The next term I want to bring to your attention is oxygen transport. Oxygen transport answers the following question: In a minute, how much oxygen leaves the heart to be delivered to the tissues? You can estimate that value by multiplying the cardiac output (in l/min) times arterial oxygen content (in ml/100 ml blood) times 10. In the example shown in Figure 5, if the patient's cardiac output is 5 l/min and arterial oxygen content is 18 ml/100 ml blood, then every minute 900 ml of oxygen leaves the heart to be delivered to the tissues.

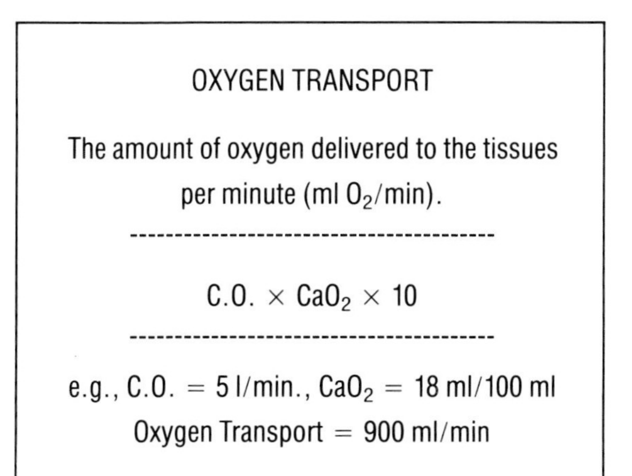

Figure 5

The final term I want to redefine today is oxygen consumption before we move on to consider some aspects of physiology. Oxygen consumption answers the following question: In a minute, how much oxygen is consumed by the body's tissues? If you know the amount of oxygen delivered to the tissues from the heart, arterial oxygen transport, and subtract from that the amount of oxygen that returns from the tissues back to the heart, venous oxygen transport, clearly the difference will be the amount of oxygen consumed by the tissues. We remember that you can represent transport as ten times cardiac output times arterial content; and venous transport as ten times cardiac output times venous content. Factor out the ten as cardiac output, and you come to this very familiar expression: Oxygen consumption is ten times cardiac output times A-V oxygen content difference, as illustrated in Figure 6. Remember, we can estimate content by simply considering the amount combined with hemoglobin and ignoring the amount dissolved. That introduces only a trivial error. Therefore, oxygen consumption can be expressed as: Cardiac output times the hemoglobin times 13.8 times the A-V saturation difference.

O_2 CONSUMPTION (ml O_2/min)

$$\text{Arterial } O_2 \text{ Transport} - \text{Venous } O_2 \text{ Transport}$$
$$10 \times C.O. \times CaO_2 - 10 \times C.O. \times C\bar{v}O_2$$
$$10 \times C.O. \times (CaO_2 - C\bar{v}O_2)$$
$$10 \times C.O. \times$$
$$(Hb \times 1.38 \times SaO_2) - (Hb \times 1.38 \times S\bar{v}O_2)$$
$$C.O. \times Hb \times 13.8 \times (SaO_2 - S\bar{v}O_2)$$

Figure 6

If you search for a unifying factor in critically ill patients (patients in shock, whether it is hemorrhagic, septic or cardiogenic), you will find in the literature that lactic acidosis is a common feature. Regardless of the type of shock, when a patient is in end-stage serious shock with an ominous prognosis the blood lactate is almost invariably elevated.

The blood lactate is elevated because the body's oxygen demands are not being met by the oxygen delivery system. In normal people the oxygen consumption must be equal to demand. When that occurs there is no lactic acidosis. When consumption is less than demand in the various types of shock, as shown in Figure 7, lactic acidosis results. Then, unless you can intervene, death will quickly follow.

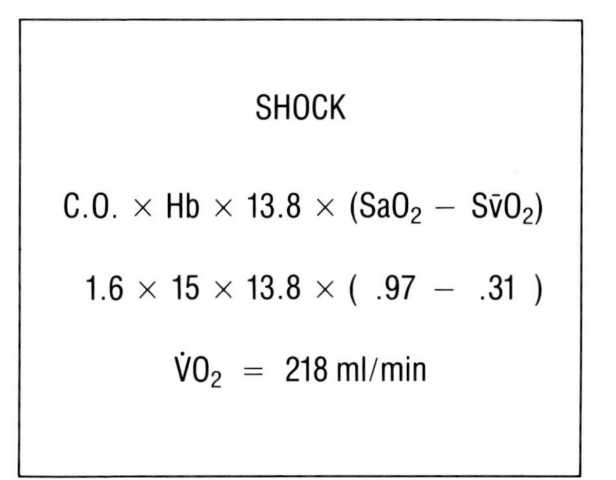

Figure 7

Let us look at some normal values for oxygen consumption. With a cardiac output of 5 l/min, a hemoglobin of 15 gm/dl, arterial saturation of 97% and a venous saturation of 75% (all normal values) the oxygen consumption is approximately 228 ml/min, as shown in Figure 8.

NORMAL

$$C.O. \times Hb \times 13.8 \times (SaO_2 - S\bar{v}O_2)$$

$$5 \times 15 \times 13.8 \times (.97 - .75)$$

$$\dot{V}O_2 = 228 \text{ ml/min}$$

Figure 8

Weil's group at U.S.C. showed in patients with myocardial infarction resulting from cardiogenic shock, that as the lactate increases (as the patient's oxygen consumption fails to meet tissue oxygen demand) prognosis is dismal.

If we understand that the expression shown in Figure 9 is oxygen consumption; and we understand that it is up to the oxygen delivery system to make sure that oxygen consumption equals demand, we can now ask ourselves two questions. First, in the critically ill patient, what are the factors that can threaten the value of this expression? The three major factors are: A decrease in cardiac output, a decrease in hemoglobin, and a fall in arterial saturation. We will deal with these systematically, shortly.

$$C.O. \times Hb \times 13.8 \times (Sa0_2 - S\bar{v}0_2)$$

Figure 9

Before we look at the factors that can threaten the value of this expression, let us ask ourselves a second question: What are the compensatory steps the body can take when the value of this expression is threatened? These compensatory steps will turn out to be very important in the critically ill patient. There are two fundamental steps the body can take. It can increase cardiac output, or by extracting more oxygen from capillary blood, it can decrease $S\bar{v}O_2$.

When athletes exercise they can actually quintuple their cardiac output, increasing it from 5 l/min all the way up to 25 l/min. Most of us can at least triple our cardiac output.

On the other hand, if we look at oxygen extraction as in Figure 10, the normal $S\bar{v}O_2$ is 75% and the normal A-V saturation difference with an arterial saturation of 97% is 22%. When a normal individual is exercising, $S\bar{v}O_2$ can decrease all the way down to 31%, thereby increasing A-V saturation difference from 22% to 66%. Once more, a factor of three.

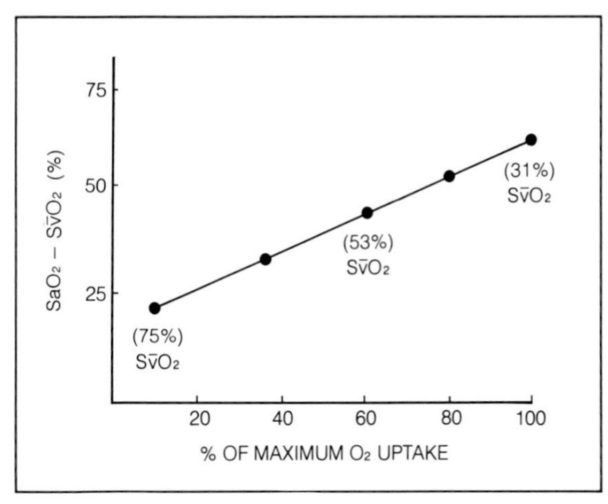

Figure 10

Normal individuals can increase their cardiac output by a factor of three and increase their A-V saturation difference by a factor of three. If you look at athletes and maximum oxygen consumption, by tripling cardiac output and by tripling the A-V saturation difference from 22% to 66%, an exercising man or woman can increase oxygen consumption by some nine-fold, as shown in Figure 11. Indeed, some athletes can do more.

MAXIMUM O_2 CONSUMPTION

$$C.O. \times Hb \times 13.8 \times (SaO_2 - S\bar{v}O_2)$$

$$15 \times 15 \times 13.8 \times (.97 - .31)$$

2049 ml/min

Figure 11

We are not here today to discuss what steps athletes take to increase their oxygen consumption. However, these same compensatory mechanisms are used by critically ill patients in intensive care units.

Now, let us return to looking systematically at this expression of oxygen consumption, and go through the factors that can threaten the value of this expression.

First, a decrease in hemoglobin. I would hope that you would agree with me that there is no question if hemoglobin falls, that the value of this expression will decrease. Then, the body must take steps to compensate for the fall in hemoglobin to prevent consumption from falling below the demand and to prevent the ominous development of lactic acidosis.

Patients with anemia have a high cardiac output as they attempt to keep consumption equal to demand. In fact, you can decrease hemoglobin from the normal 15 gm/dl to 1.6 gm/dl; but if you triple cardiac output and you maximally desaturate venous blood, oxygen consumption will remain normal, as shown in Figure 12. That observation underlies the clinical axiom that you do not see lactic acidosis in uncomplicated anemia. Patients can compensate all the way down to a hemoglobin of 1.6 gm/dl. Clearly, patients with hemoglobins of 4, 5, and 6 will not develop lactic acidosis as long as nothing else is going on.

ANEMIA

$$C.O. \times Hb \times 13.8 \times (SaO_2 - S\bar{v}O_2)$$

$$15 \times 1.6 \times 13.8 \times (.97 - .31)$$

$$\dot{V}O_2 = 218 \text{ ml/min}$$

Figure 12

How about arterial saturation? There is no question that a fall in arterial saturation will threaten the value of this expression. There is no question that the body must take steps; and, in fact, it does. If someone's saturation falls all the way down from 97% to 38% (once again a remarkable fall in arterial saturation), and the patient triples cardiac output and maximally desaturates mixed capillary blood, oxygen consumption remains normal, as shown in Figure 13. This observation underlies the second clinical axiom: In uncomplicated arterial hypoxemia, you do not get lactic acidosis.

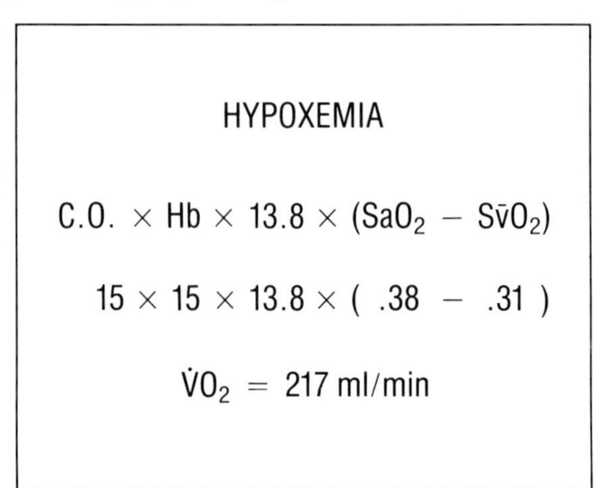

Figure 13

We all have patients with chronic lung disease, who run PO_2 levels of 35 mm Hg, with arterial oxygen saturations of 65% to 70%. They do not develop lactic acidosis unless something else is going on. Clearly, if the arterial PO_2 goes low enough, you can exhaust the compensatory mechanisms. But, by and large, do not expect to see lactic acidosis with the kinds of hypoxemia we see clinically. Or, perhaps expressed in a different way, if you do see lactic acidosis in someone with a PO_2 of 40 mmHg or 45 mmHg, you cannot explain it by the hypoxemia you are observing. Figure 14 demonstrates that. Two years ago a 70 year old man came in with respiratory failure. He had a chronic respiratory disease just at a point where the PO_2 was 19 and the lactate was normal. Hypoxemia alone does not cause lactic acidosis.

HYPOXEMIA ALONE DOES NOT CAUSE LACTIC ACIDOSIS		
70 Year Old Male With Respiratory Failure		
pH	=	7.29
pCO_2 (mm Hg)	=	64
PO_2 (mm Hg)	=	19
HCO_3 (mEq/l)	=	30
Lactate (mmol/l)	=	0.9

Figure 14

We have seen that the body has excellent compensatory mechanisms to cope with decreases in hemoglobin and arterial saturation. We are left with the final threat to oxygen consumption—a decrease in cardiac output. A decrease in cardiac output is qualitatively different than a decrease in hemoglobin or arterial saturation. Why? A fall in cardiac output not only threatens the value of this expression in the same way that anemia and arterial desaturation do, but it also eliminates one of the major compensatory mechanisms. Therefore, instead of being left with a nine-fold safety margin as you have with anemia or arterial desaturation, you are left with a three-fold safety margin. The only compensatory steps the body can take when cardiac output falls is to extract more oxygen and decrease $S\bar{v}O_2$.

Before thermodilution cardiac output was easily available in the ICU environment, $S\bar{v}O_2$ was called a "poor-man's cardiac output". When cardiac output decreased, $S\bar{v}O_2$ fell. Looking at that relationship the other way, if a decrease in $S\bar{v}O_2$ with a normal arterial saturation and hemoglobin was found, it meant cardiac output was low, as shown in Figure 15.

CAUSES OF ↓ $S\bar{v}O_2$

1. Anemia
2. Low Cardiac Output
3. Arterial Oxygen Desaturation
4. ↑ Oxygen Consumption

Figure 15

With anemia and arterial desaturation a normal person can tolerate a tremendous decrease in these values as compared to normal. However, once cardiac output has decreased to one-third of its normal value the one compensatory mechanism available has been exhausted, and lactic acidosis will occur. Perfusion failure probably remains the most common cause of lactic acidosis in a clinical setting.

ACRONYMS

$A\text{-}VO_2$ arterial-venous oxygen difference
CaO_2 arterial oxygen content
CO_2 blood oxygen content
C.O. cardiac output
$C\bar{v}O_2$ mixed venous oxygen content
Hb hemoglobin
HbO_2 oxyhemoglobin
$M\dot{V}O_2$ myocardial oxygen consumption
PaO_2 arterial oxygen pressure
PO_2 oxygen pressure
SaO_2 arterial oxygen saturation
SO_2 oxygen saturation
$S\bar{v}O_2$ mixed venous oxygen saturation
$\dot{V}O_2$ oxygen consumption

CLINICAL EXPERIENCE WITH CONTINUOUS MONITORING OF MIXED VENOUS OXYGEN SATURATION IN RESPIRATORY FAILURE

2

Patrick J. Fahey, M.D.*

The objective of my presentation is to share with you some of our experiences with continuous measurement of mixed venous oxygen saturation ($S\bar{v}O_2$), particularly those cases in which we found it to be a most helpful monitoring device. As a pulmonary physician, I have been a rather poor monitor of a patient's condition. Instead, I have been an avid tester, sending many tests to the laboratory and receiving results back. These tests, however, have provided information only at a single point in time, which may or may not be reliable or predictive of future events. Until now, we have not had technology available that allowed for continuous monitoring of a critically ill patient's physiologic status.

I continue to be surprised and impressed by the information supplied through continuous measurement of venous oxygen levels. To illustrate the value of this technological innovation as an aid in the therapy of critically ill patients, I will discuss a study in which we used $S\bar{v}O_2$ values as a method of titrating positive end-expiratory pressure (PEEP) in patients with acute hypoxemic respiratory failure.

*Associate Professor of Medicine
Loyola University Medical Center
Maywood, Illinois 50153

As shown in Figure 1, when you remove a patient from mechanical ventilation to perform endotracheal suctioning, arterial oxygen saturation frequently falls. We have been impressed that the declines in $S\bar{v}O_2$ frequently outdistance the observed falls in arterial O_2 levels. If we simultaneously placed an ear oximeter on a patient during endotracheal suctioning, we frequently saw declines in arterial saturation of 5% to 10%, while simultaneously recorded $S\bar{v}O_2$ levels declined 10%, 15%, or even 20%. Clearly, changes in arterial saturation are only the tip of the desaturation iceberg during suctioning of a patient on mechanical ventilation.

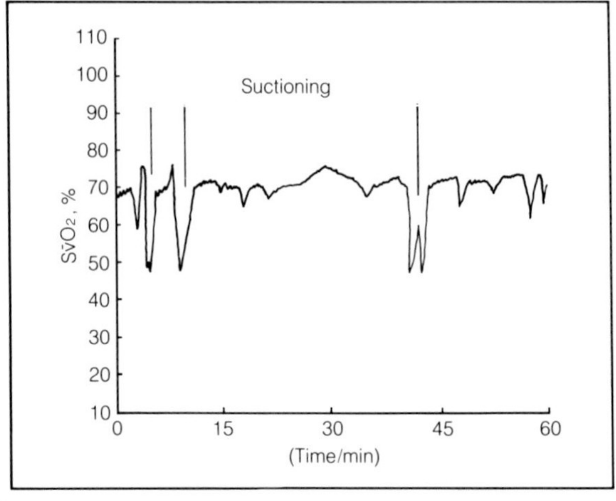

Figure 1
Fall in $S\bar{v}O_2$ during endotracheal suctioning.

To more precisely document the cause of declines in $S\bar{v}O_2$ during endotracheal suctioning, we measured cardiac output in three patients before and during the suctioning period. In two patients, cardiac output increased more than 25%, with an associated increase in O_2 consumption of over 40%! This marked rise in O_2 consumption most likely represented the energy requirements associated with coughing and agitation that were induced by irritation of the airways by the catheter tip. In one patient, we observed a fall in cardiac output from 5.2 to 3.8 L/min associated with suctioning, while O_2 consumption remained essentially unchanged. Thus, endotracheal suctioning of critically ill mechanically ventilated patients carries a physiologic stress. This stress is only partially appreciated by measurement of arterial oxygen levels, but it is most dramatically seen by changes in $S\bar{v}O_2$. The large changes in $S\bar{v}O_2$

are frequently due to increased oxygen demands of tissues outstripping O_2 supply. In addition, some patients appear to have declines in cardiac output associated with endotracheal suctioning.

The cough mechanism has been called the watchdog of the lung. Sometimes, however, the watchdog is too vigilant and irritable. Figure 2 shows a 65-year-old gentleman in the throes of chronic, refractory congestive heart failure, requiring 60% oxygen by face mask to establish 90% arterial O_2 saturation. He had repeated and protracted coughing spasms that we felt were due to irritant receptor stimulation secondary to increased hydrostatic pressure in his pulmonary interstitium. During many of these coughing spells we noted repeated decreases in $S\bar{v}O_2$ to as low as 40%. Simultaneous measurement of his arterial saturation during these episodes showed no significant change. Why would $S\bar{v}O_2$ dip so low during coughing?

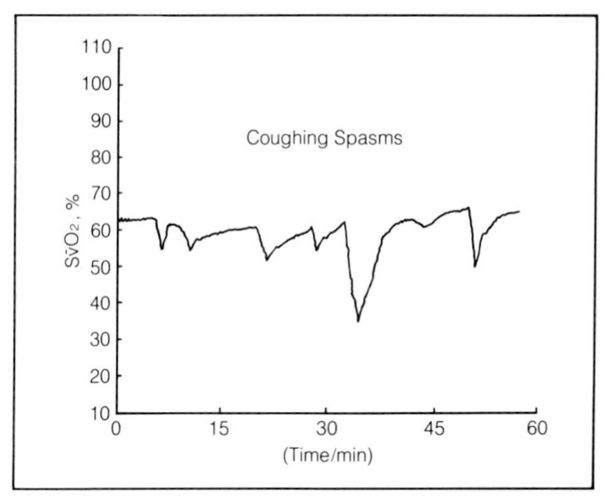

Figure 2
Fall in $S\bar{v}O_2$ during coughing in chronic, refractory congestive heart failure.

To further elucidate this problem, we measured cardiac output before and during a protracted coughing episode and found that not only had the cardiac output decreased, but O_2 consumption had risen more than 30%. We suspect that the Valsalva maneuver involved during coughing increased intrathoracic pressure sufficiently to decrease venous return and this led to the fall in cardiac output. In addition, the increased oxygen demands of the respiratory muscles involved in coughing led to profound desaturation of the venous blood.

Such changes have alerted us to be more aggressive in sedating anxious patients and in attempting to suppress chronic and distressing cough, particularly in patients with associated cardiac disease in whom routine activities such as coughing, suctioning, and changing position represent severe physiologic stresses.

Figure 3 illustrates a case frequently seen in our ICU. This patient had respiratory failure secondary to advanced chronic obstructive pulmonary disease (COPD), along with evidence of fluid overload and pulmonary edema due to left ventricular failure. Despite aggressive medical management, he progressed to respiratory failure with hypoxemia and had to be intubated. He required an inspired oxygen concentration (FIO_2) of 50%, 10 cm H_2O of PEEP, and synchronous intermittent mandatory ventilation (SIMV) at a rate of 12 to maintain an adequate arterial oxygen level and PCO_2. When he had not made satisfactory progress after three days, we inserted an Opticath® to assess his hemodynamic status. We were immediately struck by the low $S\bar{v}O_2$ value of near 50% that we initially encountered. At this time, the patient was breathing in the SIMV mode with a respiratory rate of 28 breaths/min and a mandatory rate of 12/min. My initial suspicion was that cardiac output must be decreased to account for such a low $S\bar{v}O_2$. Therefore, I tried a short period of spontaneous breathing with the pressure support mode of ventilation. In this mode, the patient breathed spontaneously, and inspiratory gas flow was supplemented to a preset positive pressure to decrease the inherent resistance in the ventilator and associated tubings.

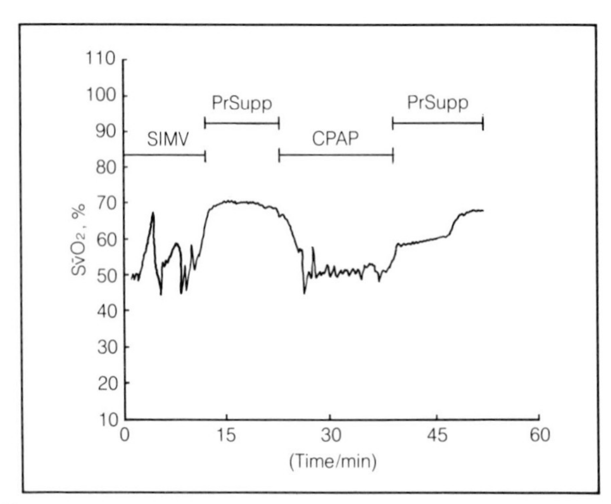

Figure 3
Continuous $S\bar{v}O_2$ monitoring in a patient with respiratory failure and hypoxemia.

As you can see, there was an immediate and dramatic rise in $S\bar{v}O_2$ to near normal levels of 70% associated with the change in ventilator mode. Arterial oxygen levels did not change, nor did cardiac output. We compared oxygen consumption, using the Fick equation, between SIMV and pressure support mode of ventilation and found an almost 47% decrease in oxygen consumption when this patient was breathing with pressure support.

Under healthy circumstances, the respiratory muscles account for approximately 5% of total oxygen consumption, making it a very energy efficient system. However, when we measured oxygen consumption in patients with respiratory failure, we frequently found the oxygen cost of breathing approached 25% to 30% of total O_2 consumption. Thus, in many patients with respiratory failure, mechanical ventilation can be of significant benefit because it may reduce the oxygen cost of breathing. In addition, we have found that the mode of ventilation may also be important, particularly in patients with alterations in lung compliance and resistance. While I have been a proponent of the advantages of SIMV compared to assist-control ventilation, we have found that oxygen consumption increased significantly in some patients when they were breathing in SIMV mode. Because of this, I have reassessed my loyalty to this mode of ventilation. Alternatively, we have occasionally found patients with higher $S\bar{v}O_2$ levels when they were breathing in the SIMV mode compared to assist-control. These changes seem likely to be due to improvement of cardiac output. The availability of continuous $S\bar{v}O_2$ has given us a sensitive indicator of the appropriateness of our mode of ventilation and status of O_2 consumption in patients requiring mechanical ventilation.

I will now present an interesting case that led to evaluation of the role of $S\bar{v}O_2$ in the titration of PEEP therapy. Figure 4 is the tracing of a 25-year-old male factory worker who complained of the sudden onset of headache at work followed by his collapse. When brought to our emergency room, he was in severe respiratory distress, with fluid bubbling out of his mouth. Though intubated, his arterial PO_2 was only 47 mm Hg on 100% oxygen. He required 15 cm H_2O of PEEP to increase his PO_2 to 84 mm Hg. While intubated, he was taken to the radiology department for a computed axial tomography (CT) scan of the head, which showed a large intracerebral hemorrhage. We believed he was suffering from neurogenic pulmonary edema, and he was started on both mannitol and dexamethasone in an attempt to decrease cerebral edema. When transferred to the medical ICU, the chest film in this previously healthy 260 lb man showed fluffy bilateral alveolar infiltrates with a normal heart size. We placed a pulmonary artery catheter in him because, generally, I am uncomfortable with the hemodynamic status of patients requiring more than 15 cm H_2O of PEEP. Pulmonary capillary wedge pressure was 8 mm Hg, confirming the noncardiac nature of the pulmonary edema.

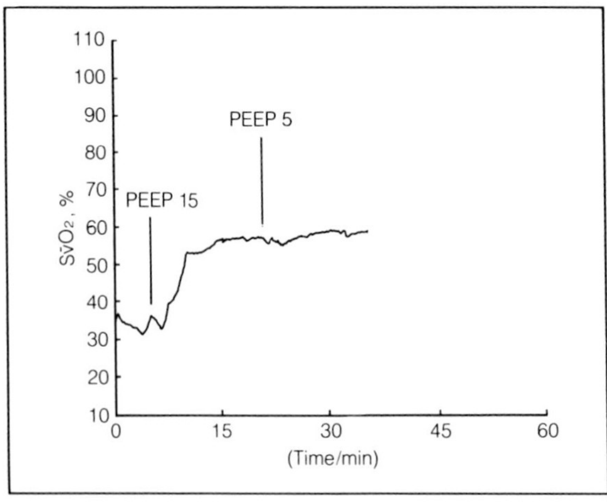

Figure 4

Decreasing PEEP led to an increase in $S\bar{v}O_2$ in a patient with severe respiratory distress.

The initial $S\bar{v}O_2$ was quite low at 38% saturation; an arterial PO_2 collected at the same time was 68 mm Hg. While taking some comfort from the normal level of arterial oxygen, I was distressed to see the venous oxygen so low. I decided to see what would happen if I decreased the PEEP, all the time thinking I could not make the situation much worse. Following decrease in PEEP to 5 cm H_2O, there was a prompt increase in $S\bar{v}O_2$ from below 40% to near 60%. Interestingly, at the same time arterial PO_2 decreased to 51 mm Hg.

At first glance, it seemed a paradoxical situation. Despite evidence of improved tissue oxygenation as detected by the large increase in $S\bar{v}O_2$, we were faced with decreasing arterial oxygen levels following the decrease in PEEP. I suspect that cardiac output was quite low when he was initially transferred to our ICU. The mannitol therapy had resulted in more than a 4-L diuresis in a two-hour period, most likely leaving his intravascular fluid volume depleted and making the untoward effects of PEEP therapy that much greater. Thus, the decrease in PEEP likely augmented his venous return and cardiac output. Despite the decline in arterial oxygen content, oxygen delivery to the tissues was enhanced overall.

Such abrupt and dynamic changes in venous oxygen levels are not supposed to occur in patients with adult respiratory distress syndrome (ARDS), (Danek et al: American Review of Respiratory Disease, 122:387-395, 1980). They reported that the venous oxygen levels often did not change despite large changes in cardiac output in ARDS patients. This was believed to be due to a change in oxygen consumption associated with a change in oxygen delivery (i.e., that O_2 consumption was dependent on O_2 delivery). Our clinical experience has been quite different, as this case of neurogenic pulmonary edema illustrates. We found that venous oxygen levels, in fact, vary widely and dynamically during the course of ARDS and particularly with changes in therapy. We decided to undertake a more rigorous study of the relationship between $S\bar{v}O_2$ and oxygen delivery in patients requiring PEEP therapy as a result of acute hypoxemic respiratory failure.

Thus far, we have studied eight patients. Etiologies of respiratory failure reflected the "mixed bag" type of patients we see in our medical ICU. Underlying conditions included Goodpasture's syndrome, postarrest congestive heart failure, pneumonia, cirrhosis, and an anaphylactic reaction associated with administration of platelets. Two patients were septic. The patient with cirrhosis developed spontaneous bacterial peritonitis with *Escherichia coli* in his blood. One patient with staphylococcal pnuemonia was also septic. The average FIO_2 was 0.60 and the average PO_2 64 mm Hg. All required PEEP between 5 and 10 cm H_2O. To enter the study, we required that each patient be hemodynamically stable and relaxed, which often required sedation. A non anxious patient was important because we had been impressed by large changes in oxygen consumption that can occur when a patient is fighting the ventilator, reacting to increased PEEP, or is generally apprehensive about being in an ICU on a ventilator. We've become far more aggressive in our use of sedation in our patients requiring PEEP therapy. Each patient was placed on 5, 10, 15, or 20 cm H_2O of PEEP for 25 minutes. We then determined cardiac output and arterial and mixed venous oxygen levels. From these measurements, we determined oxygen delivery at each level of PEEP and correlated the $S\bar{v}O_2$ at that point.

Figure 5 shows the change in $S\bar{v}O_2$ associated with each level of PEEP. Each point represents the mean of eight patients, ±1 standard deviation. As PEEP was increased, $S\bar{v}O_2$ declined in seven of the eight patients. The fall in $S\bar{v}O_2$ is related to a significant decrease in cardiac output, which occurred in six of the eight patients. As PEEP was increased from 5 to 20 cm H_2O, $S\bar{v}O_2$ declined from 72% to 62% saturation as shown in Figure 6. There was a strong, intrasubject correlation between changes in $S\bar{v}O_2$ and oxygen delivery.

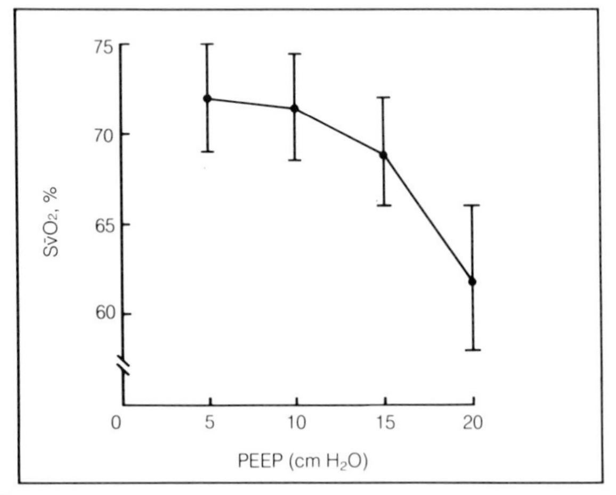

Figure 5
Changes in $S\bar{v}O_2$ associated with changes in the level of PEEP.

In seven of eight patients, the highest level of $S\bar{v}O_2$ identified the highest oxygen delivery. The one patient for whom there was no correlation had staphylococcal sepsis, while the patient with *E. coli* sepsis showed a strong correlation between changes in O_2 delivery and $S\bar{v}O_2$. Figure 7 is a graph of the individual data from each of the eight patients with $S\bar{v}O_2$ versus oxygen delivery. In six of eight patients, there was strong correlation between $S\bar{v}O_2$ and O_2 delivery.

PEEP (cm H_2O)	$S\bar{v}O_2$, %	O_2 DELIVERY (ml/min)
5	72 ± 6	905 ± 274
10	71 ± 5	873 ± 256
15	69 ± 6	834 ± 248
20	62 ± 10	726 ± 312

Figure 6
Relationship between amounts of PEEP, $S\bar{v}O_2$, and oxygen delivery.

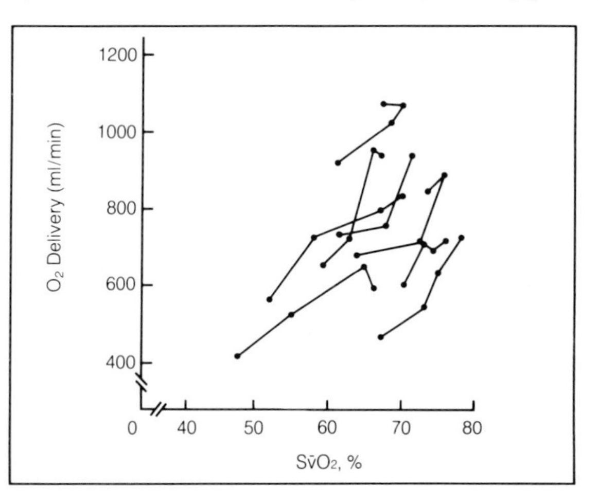

Figure 7
Correlation between $S\bar{v}O_2$ and O_2 delivery.

In this preliminary investigation, we have begun to appreciate the value of $S\bar{v}O_2$ as a monitoring device in the ICU for detecting unsuspected episodes of threatened tissue oxygenation and as a method for titrating PEEP therapy.

USE OF CONTINUOUS MONITORING OF MIXED VENOUS OXYGEN SATURATION IN THE MANAGEMENT OF MECHANICAL VENTILATION FOR RESPIRATORY FAILURE

3

John C. McMichan, M.B., B.S., Ph.D.*

The amount of oxygen attached to hemoglobin in pulmonary arterial blood is a reflection of cardiopulmonary function and tissue oxygen consumption. These factors are related by the Fick equation, which can be rewritten as follows:

$$S\bar{v}O_2 = SaO_2 - \frac{\dot{V}O_2}{Q_T \times Hb \times 1.34}$$

where $S\bar{v}O_2$ is the mixed venous oxygen saturation, SaO_2 is the arterial oxygen saturation, $\dot{V}O_2$ is the oxygen consumption, Q_T is the cardiac output, and Hb is the concentration of hemoglobin. It is apparent from this equation that $S\bar{v}O_2$ is directly proportional to SaO_2, Q_T, and Hb and inversely proportional to $\dot{V}O_2$. In the acute situation, it is unusual for the hemoglobin concentration to change rapidly; therefore, a decrease in $S\bar{v}O_2$ will generally result from a decrease in pulmonary (SaO_2) or cardiac function (Q_T), or from an increase in the utilization of oxygen by the tissues ($\dot{V}O_2$). Thus, $S\bar{v}O_2$ can be used to interpret changes in pulmonary function if cardiac

*Director of Surgical and Respiratory ICU
Department of Anesthesia
Mayo Clinic
Rochester, Minnesota 55905

factors and oxygen consumption remain constant. Similarly, it can reflect changes in cardiac function if oxygen consumption and pulmonary function remain the same. These are artificial circumstances not often seen in clinical practice. However, oxygen consumption can be considered stable in the anesthetized and paralyzed patient so that under the conditions of anesthesia, mixed venous oxygen saturation provides a close reflection of cardiopulmonary function. In the intensive care setting, this relationship is not as close. Nevertheless, by observing the patient for obvious changes in oxygen consumption (e.g., restlessness), a good estimate of the stability of cardiopulmonary function can be obtained by observing the changes in $S\bar{v}O_2$.

The aim of cardiopulmonary function is to supply oxygen to the tissues. This supply can be defined as oxygen delivery, which is the product of arterial oxygen content (CaO_2) and cardiac output. Oxygen delivery usually satisfies demand ($\dot{V}O_2$), but when this balance fails, extra oxygen is made available to the tissues by alterations in Q_T, CaO_2, or by increases in oxygen extraction from the blood. In the acute situation, increased oxygen demand is met initially by increases in cardiac output. When cardiac output cannot increase sufficiently to meet the increased demand, oxygen extraction increases and the amount of oxygen remaining in mixed venous blood decreases. Thus, monitoring of $S\bar{v}O_2$ provides feedback of changes occurring in cardiopulmonary function or tissue oxygen consumption.

This feedback can be of considerable value in the intensive care setting if the response time of the monitoring system is short and the system is able to respond to a rapidly changing variable. This is indeed the case with the OXIMETRIX® Opticath® Oximetry System,[1] so a continuous measurement of $S\bar{v}O_2$ is available at the bedside when factors affecting respiratory function are altered over a short space of time. The combination of accurate measurement and rapid response time permits an almost immediate feedback of the effects of alterations in respiratory support in the presence of acute respiratory failure.

Among the important characteristics of mechanical ventilation are the inspired oxygen fraction (FIO_2), the mode of mechanical ventilation, and the use of positive end-expiratory pressure (PEEP). When commencing mechanical ventilation, the value of FIO_2, the need for assisted, controlled, intermittent mandatory (IMV), or other modes of ventilation, and the use of PEEP are determined, and then their effects are observed on hemodynamic parameters and arterial blood gas tensions. In the presence of continuous $S\bar{v}O_2$ monitoring, the effects of these characteristics can be observed long before hemodynamic variables can be measured or arterial blood gases analyzed. For example, a change in mode of mechanical ventilation from assist-control to IMV, which results in improved ventilation-perfusion matching and oxygen delivery, will produce either a stable or an increasing level of $S\bar{v}O_2$, indicating that such a ventilator change was appropriate.

The use of PEEP to improve oxygenation and thus permit a decrease in FIO_2 is of benefit as long as cardiac function is not compromised at the same time. If PEEP increases CaO_2 without decreasing Q_T, oxygen delivery will improve. However, for each patient at a particular level of cardiac preload, there is a point at which PEEP will begin to decrease cardiac output and therefore decrease oxygen delivery.[2] As PEEP increases toward this value, oxygen delivery may increase (as CaO_2 increases), and $S\bar{v}O_2$ will increase or remain constant. When this value is exceeded, oxygen delivery will begin to decrease (because cardiac output falls), and oxygen extraction will increase, producing a decrease in $S\bar{v}O_2$. Before the availability of continuous monitoring of $S\bar{v}O_2$, the determination of this value of PEEP required multiple determinations of cardiac output and arterial blood gas tensions, thus consuming both time and money. With the advent of the OXIMETRIX Opticath Oximetry System, the determination of this level of PEEP is possible without multiple measurements and significant expenditures because of the rapid response of the System to changes in PEEP.

During recovery from acute respiratory failure of a severity sufficient to require mechanical ventilation, bedside decisions are made regarding the appropriate time and degree of decrease of mechanical ventilatory support. This weaning period often begins with a change to IMV mode of the mechanical ventilator followed by either a decrease in the PEEP level or in the IMV rate. The next step usually entails a trial of spontaneous ventilation followed by extubation. The safety and correct timing of each step in this weaning process can be easily observed as soon as each step is undertaken by using the OXIMETRIX Opticath Oximetry System. Thus, inappropriate steps in the weaning procedure or too rapid advance towards extubation can be immediately detected and reversed without the patient being subjected to dangerous episodes of unobserved hypoxia.

The continuous monitoring of $S\bar{v}O_2$ becomes the "bottom line" in determining the appropriateness, the timing, and the degree of mechanical ventilator support necessary for the patient with acute respiratory failure. Its rapid response time provides early warning for the physician to take appropriate steps to reverse this trend. A decrease in $S\bar{v}O_2$ will not necessarily indicate which system failure is involved, but it will stimulate appropriate investigations of cardiopulmonary function if there is time, or in the extremely acute situation, it will indicate the response to therapeutic modalities chosen on an empirical basis.

REFERENCES

1. Baele, P.L., McMichan, J.C., Marsh, H.M., Sill, J.C., Southorn, P.A.: Continuous monitoring of mixed venous oxygen saturation in critically ill patients. Anesth. Analg. 61:513-517, 1982.
2. Suter, P.M., Fairley, H.B., Isenberg, M.D.: Optimum end-expiratory airway pressure in patients with acute pulmonary failure. N. Engl. J. Med. 292:284-289, 1975.

CLINICAL USEFULNESS OF CONTINUOUS MONITORING OF MIXED VENOUS OXYGEN SATURATION

4

Paul M. Stevens, M.D.*

Intermittent sampling of arterial blood gas tensions has been the accepted method of monitoring oxygenation for nearly 20 years. However, it is becoming increasingly obvious that there is little relationship between arterial O_2 tension (PaO_2) and prognosis for survival.[1]

Arterial gas tensions reflect the efficiency of ventilation and gas exchange in the lungs. Similarly, the measurement of venous blood gases reflects the oxygen tension at the end of the capillary of the tissue it supplies. Unfortunately, there are many organs of interest whose venous effluent make up the mixed venous blood sample obtained from the pulmonary artery. Thus, this sample reflects only generally the overall status of the body's oxygen demand.

The relationship of the mixed venous O_2 content ($C\bar{v}O_2$) to the body's oxygenation status is derived from the well-known and time-proven Fick equation.[2] When rewritten, this principle states that the oxygen consumption of the body ($\dot{V}O_2$) is a function of the cardiac output (C.O.) and the extraction of oxygen from arterial to venous blood (arterial-venous oxygen content difference or $CaO_2 - CvO_2$).

*Professor of Medicine
Baylor College of Medicine
Houston, Texas 01605

Under most normal circumstances, it has been demonstrated that the $CaO_2 - CvO_2$ is protected and remains more constant than either the cardiac output or the oxygen consumption in resting humans.[3] Thus, there are only two major determinants of $C\bar{v}O_2$: the oxygen consumption and the cardiac output. Should the oxygen consumption increase, an immediate increase in the cardiac output would result. Should the cardiac output be unable to increase for some pathological reason, compensation would take place in the form of an increase in the $CaO_2 - CvO_2$. Both mechanisms are activated to some variable degree in healthy subjects. Only under certain circumstances, however, such as exercise or environmental hypoxia, is the $C\bar{v}O_2$ maximally reduced.

In critically ill patients who are inactive, the major causes of changing cardiac output and oxygen consumption are the pathological processes that are occurring. These processes primarily affect the oxygen demand of the body. A compensatory response is achieved either through an increase in the cardiac output or a widening of the $CaO_2 - CvO_2$. When the cardiac output is unable to respond, and the arterial O_2 content is optimal, the venous oxygen content may decrease below minimum levels necessary to insure adequate tissue oxygenation.

It is important to note that oxygen consumption at the mitochondrial level requires an oxygen tension of only 1 or 2 mm Hg; therefore, there is virtually no oxygen storage. Any decrease in the O_2 gradient between the perfusing capillary and the mitochondria will further decrease the availability of O_2 and lead to anaerobiosis and subsequent tissue damage. Thus, any process that results in a reduction in the content of oxygen in venous blood can potentially cause tissue hypoxia and injury. When $C\bar{v}O_2$ is reduced below certain critical levels, injury to tissues is likely to occur.

The advent of a fiberoptic catheter that can be floated into the pulmonary artery and can continuously track the saturation of blood flowing past it allows for the continuous assessment of the major determinants of mixed venous oxygen saturation ($S\bar{v}O_2$): the arterial O_2 content and the cardiac output response to tissue O_2 demand.

ASSESSMENT OF CARDIAC OUTPUT FROM $S\bar{v}O_2$

Cardiac output measurement by thermodilution technique has become a standard procedure in many critical care units. However, it should be noted that this technique has marked variability.[4] Furthermore, changes in cardiac output may be difficult to ascertain when their absolute value is very low. As shown in Figure 1, even small changes in output must be accompanied by relatively large changes in $CaO_2 - CvO_2$ when the output is low. At high cardiac outputs, because the $CaO_2 - CvO_2$ is narrow, changes are easier to measure directly rather than depending on the small associated change in $CaO_2 - CvO_2$. Most critical care situations involve corrections of low cardiac outputs and are best reflected by changes in the $CaO_2 - CvO_2$. The example shown in Figure 2 illustrates this point.

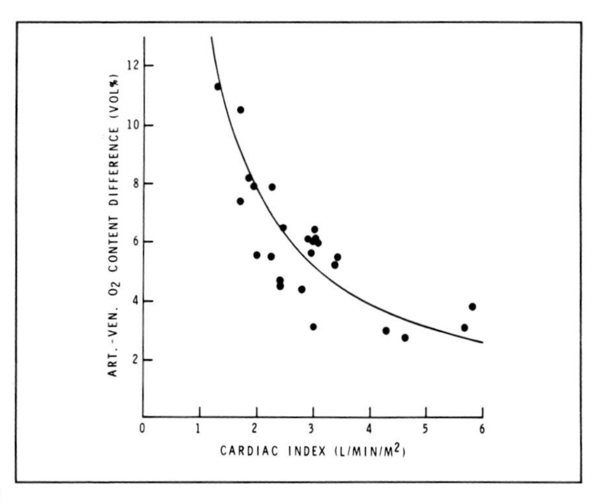

Figure 1

The relationship between cardiac index and the $CaO_2 - CvO_2$ is hyperbolic. Points represent directly measured $CaO_2 - CvO_2$ and thermodilution cardiac outputs. The curve represents the predicted oxygen consumption per square meter of body surface area for these subjects. Note how small changes in cardiac index are associated with large changes in $CaO_2 - CvO_2$ only when the index is low.

Sodium nitroprusside was being infused into this patient who had an acute myocardial infarction. All monitored parameters were in the normal range. The patient was stable and in no distress and the drip was stopped. Within ten minutes there was an abrupt fall in the previously stable $S\bar{v}O_2$, accompanied by a marked rise in the pulmonary capillary wedge and arterial pressures (PCWP, PAP). In spite of the relatively long "washout" time of the sodium nitroprusside, reinstitution resulted in the reestablishment of normal parameters within four to five minutes.

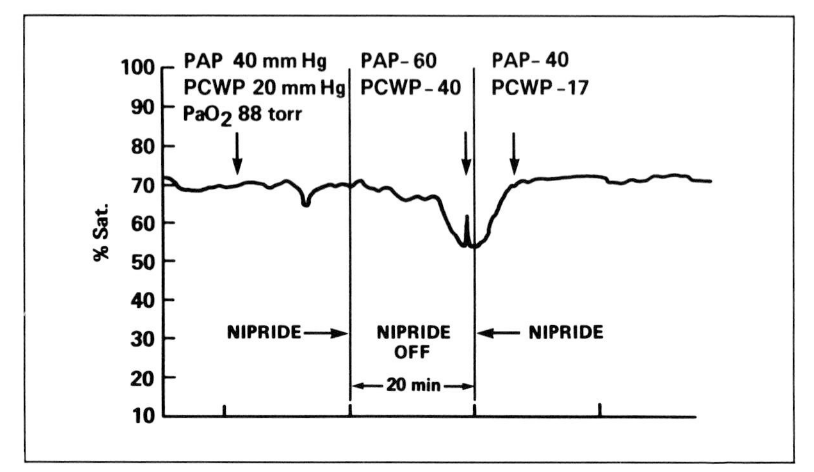

Figure 2

Cessation of sodium nitroprusside infusion is followed by a marked reduction in $S\bar{v}O_2$. This change takes approximately 15 minutes and is accompanied by a rapid increase in the PCWP. Reversal of all abnormalities occurs within five minutes of infusion resumption. The changes document the usefulness of the unloading therapy and likely reflect the changes in the cardiac output.

Progressive decrease in the $S\bar{v}O_2$ usually antedates serious hemodynamic deterioration and life-threatening events. This is illustrated in Figure 3. The clinical circumstances surrounding this event dictate whether it is due to reductions in cardiac output or arterial O_2 tension. In this example, the bradycardia likely reflected the marked reduction in coronary perfusion due to the hypotension. Atropine-induced tachycardia and its associated increase in cardiac output rapidly but transiently increased the $S\bar{v}O_2$. These observations suggest that $S\bar{v}O_2$ may be a sensitive indicator of the effect of arrhythmias on tissue oxygenation.

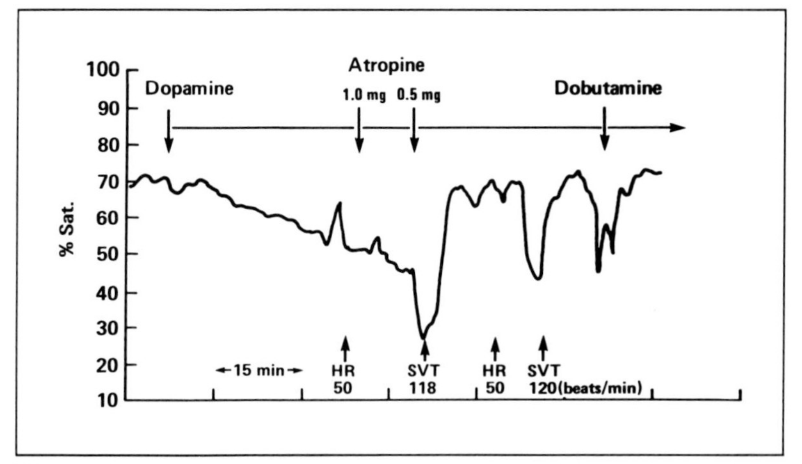

Figure 3

Gradual decline in $S\bar{v}O_2$ with onset of hypotension in a patient with acute myocardial infarction. The development of bradycardia is treated with two intravenous infusions of atropine. Supraventricular tachycardia (SVT) is accompanied by a rapid increase in $S\bar{v}O_2$, likely signifying an increase in cardiac output. A similar sequence of shorter duration is repeated. HR = heart rate.

RESPIRATOR MANAGEMENT AND $S\bar{v}O_2$

The depressant effects of positive end-expiratory pressure (PEEP) on cardiac function have been well documented.[4,5] Measurements of oxygen delivery (arterial O_2 content X cardiac output) have been recommended as a method of optimizing PEEP. However, this can be more simply achieved by monitoring the $S\bar{v}O_2$. PEEP is only justified if it results in an increase in O_2 tension or delivery. Both occurrences will result in an increase in the $S\bar{v}O_2$. Should PEEP cause either a decrease in arterial O_2 content or a reduction in cardiac output, $S\bar{v}O_2$ would be reduced. Figure 4 illustrates this point in a patient maintained on 10 cm H_2O of PEEP, which was gradually reduced with progressive increments in $S\bar{v}O_2$.

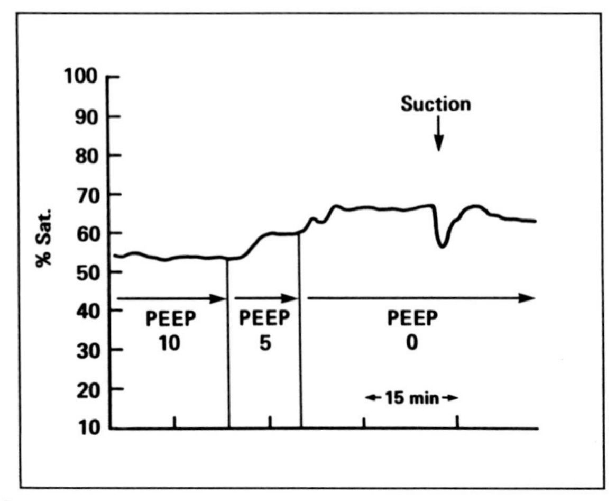

Figure 4

Patient with adult respiratory distress syndrome (ARDS) being treated with PEEP. $S\bar{v}O_2$ is marginal, and gradual reduction of PEEP is accompanied by sequential increases in $S\bar{v}O_2$, probably indicating augmentation in cardiac output previously depressed by PEEP. Note the adverse effect of suctioning.

Weaning patients who are critically ill from respirators can be a frustrating and time-consuming task. It is often difficult to determine the reasons for failure by obtrusive physical signs in the patient. Such signs include respiratory distress, tachycardia, restlessness, hypotension, etc. These signs have traditionally been thought to reflect respiratory insufficiency due to pulmonary dysfunction. Arterial blood gases, however, are often stable, and the cause of the respiratory distress is blamed on a variety of other causes such as respiratory muscle weakness, anxiety, etc. There is good experimental evidence that respiratory support can be a major factor in maintaining hemodynamic stability.[6] Continuous monitoring of $S\bar{v}O_2$ in a patient who was difficult to wean from the respirator showed dramatic reductions in saturation immediately after weaning, with no significant changes in simultaneously obtained arterial blood gas tensions.

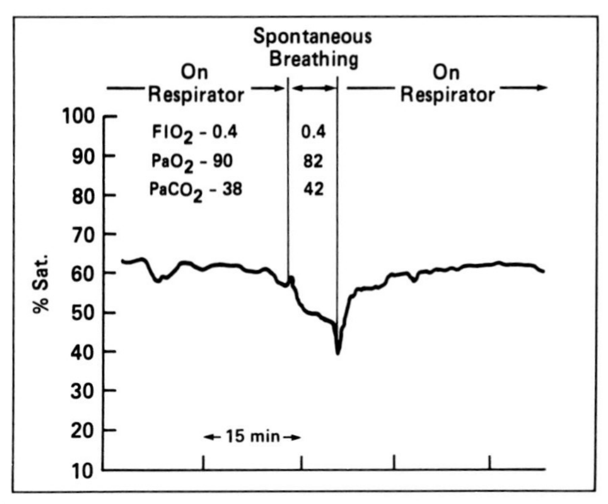

Figure 5

Weaning from respirator associated with reduction in $S\bar{v}O_2$. Spontaneous respiration causes a fall in $S\bar{v}O_2$ without appreciable change in PaO_2, indicating an increase in O_2 demand without an appropriate increase in cardiac output. FIO_2 = inspired oxygen concentration, PaO_2 = arterial oxygen tension, $PaCO_2$ = arterial carbon dioxide tension.

The cause of the reduction of $S\bar{v}O_2$ in the presence of an unchanged arterial O_2 content must be either an increase in the oxygen consumption due to the increased work of spontaneous respiration, or a failure of the cardiac output to increase in response to the increased O_2 requirements. It is possible for the cardiac output to actually decrease in response to the weaning process as exemplified in Figure 6.

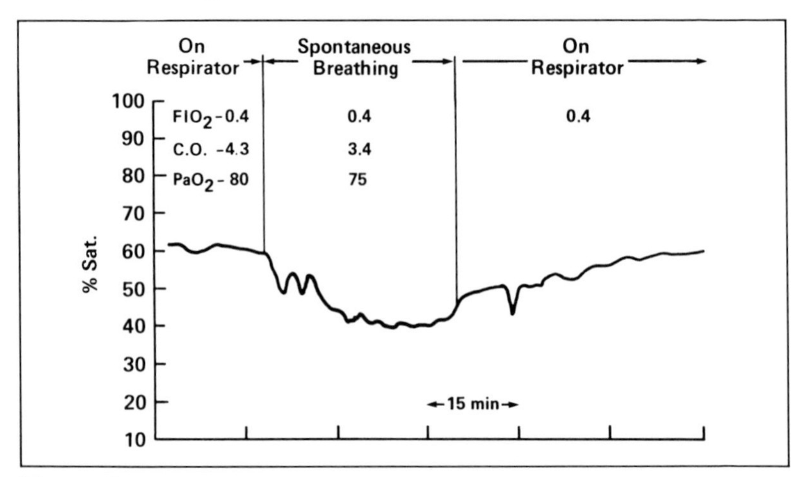

Figure 6
Poorly tolerated weaning from respirator. Reduction in $S\bar{v}O_2$ was associated with a measurable decrease in cardiac output.

The major goal of ventilatory support of the critically ill patient is the maintenance of adequate arterial oxygen tension, and this is assured through repetitive sampling of the arterial blood. Not only is this expensive, it also contributes to significant blood loss. It should be intuitively obvious that under most circumstances, stability of an adequate $S\bar{v}O_2$ must signify an adequate arterial O_2 content. Furthermore, any significant change in arterial O_2 content, and therefore tension, must be associated with some reduction in the $S\bar{v}O_2$. Even attempts to compensate for arterial hypoxemia by increasing cardiac output are likely preceded by changes in $S\bar{v}O_2$.

Continuous measurement of $S\bar{v}O_2$ allows for rapid assessment of the adequacy of arterial O_2 content in response to any respirator, mask, or inspired oxygen concentration manipulation. Thus, the FIO_2 as well as the PEEP can be changed on a respirator until a significant change in the $S\bar{v}O_2$ is achieved. Small variations in $S\bar{v}O_2$ in response to relatively large changes in the FIO_2 suggest that very little change is occurring in the arterial O_2 content and that PaO_2 is staying relatively high. However, should large changes in the $S\bar{v}O_2$ (>5%) result from changes in the FIO_2, the arterial O_2 tension must be falling to levels at which desaturation takes place. This is illustrated in Figure 7.

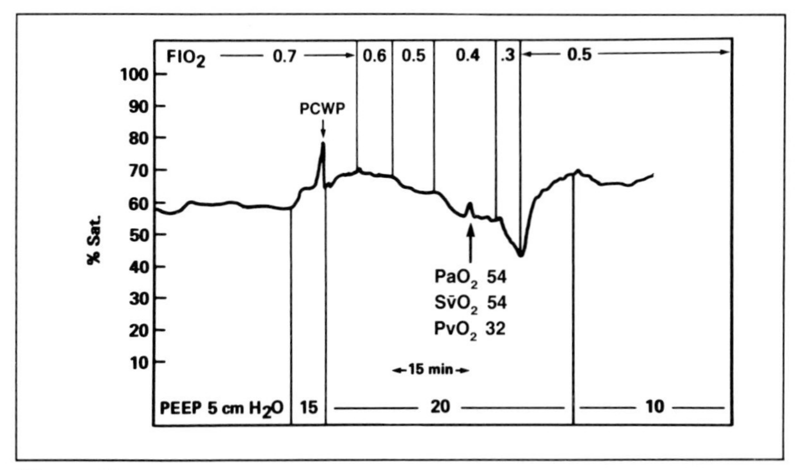

Figure 7

Regulation of FIO_2 according to changes in $S\bar{v}O_2$. Each 10% reduction in FIO_2 is accompanied by a progressively larger reduction in $S\bar{v}O_2$. This is due to reductions in PaO_2 to levels where hemoglobin desaturation occurs. Thus, one can predict from the magnitude of change in $S\bar{v}O_2$ when critical hypoxemia begins. PvO_2=venous oxygen pressure.

A patient heavily sedated and on controlled ventilation postoperatively may not respond to sudden changes in respiratory status in the expected fashion. As shown in Figure 8, previously stable $S\bar{v}O_2$ may be the only indication of dysfunction. In this example, the development of a pneumothorax was finally diagnosed because of an unexplained decrease in the $S\bar{v}O_2$. Conventionally monitored parameters changed relatively late, after the onset of the pneumothorax. In addition, the primary manifestations were hemodynamic rather than respiratory due to the circumstances under which they occurred.

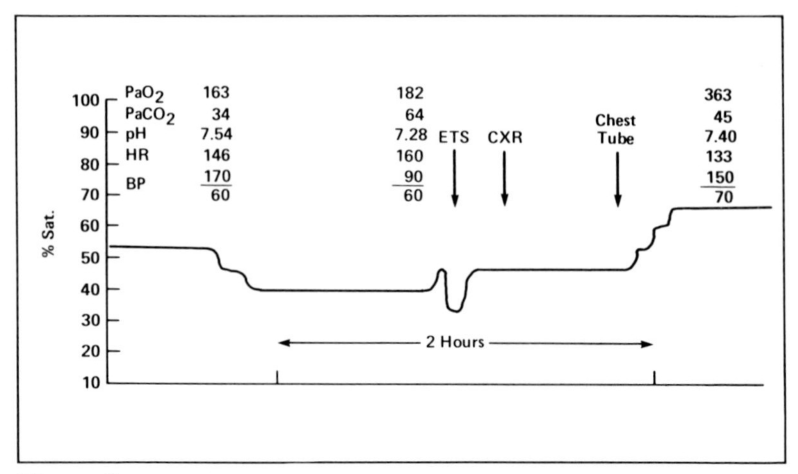

Figure 8

Unexplained reduction in $S\bar{v}O_2$ in respirator patient following thoracic aortic aneurysm resection. Onset of tachycardia and hypotension prompted measurement of arterial blood gases. CO_2 retention resulted in suctioning (ETS) with further transient reduction in $S\bar{v}O_2$. A chest film (CXR) documented the presence of a pneumothorax. Insertion of a chest tube promptly corrected the $S\bar{v}O_2$ by allowing an increase in cardiac output since arterial blood was fully saturated. BP = blood pressure.

In conclusion, $S\bar{v}O_2$ is a parameter that, if monitored, can give useful information regarding the status of oxygen transport in the critically ill patient. Changes in this value reflect changes in arterial oxygen content, cardiac output, or tissue oxygen consumption. $S\bar{v}O_2$ can now be continuously monitored with fiberoptic catheters virtually identical to those used to monitor central hemodynamics. The values obtained are reliable and accurate, and changes occur early in response to fluctuations in hemodynamics or gas exchange status. Thus, the efficacy of therapeutic interventions can be quickly assessed. The increased cost of the catheter is marginal, particularly in relationship to the savings it can provide.

REFERENCES

1. Springer R. R., Stevens P. M.: The influence of PEEP on survival in respiratory failure. Am. J. Med. 66:196-200, 1979.
2. Cournand A., et al: Measurements of cardiac output in man using technique of cardiac catheterization of the right auricle and ventricle. J. Clin. Invest. 29:106, 1945.
3. Reeves T. J., Grover R. F., Felley G. F., et al: Cardiac output in resting man. J. Appl. Physiol. 16:276-278, 1961.
4. Stetz C. W., Miller R. G., Kelly G. E., Roffin T. A.: Reliability of thermodilution method in determination of cardiac output in clinical practice. Am. Rev. Resp. Dis. 126:1001-1004, 1982.
5. Jardin F., Fargot J., Manny J.: The mechanism of depressed cardiac output on positive end expiratory pressure. N. Engl. J. Med. 304:387-392, 1981.
6. Aubier M., Viires N., Syllie G., Mozes R., Roussos C.: Respiratory muscle contributions to lactic acidosis in low cardiac output. Am. Rev. Resp. Dis. 126:648-652, 1982.
7. Divertie M. B., McMichan J. C.: Continuous monitoring of mixed venous oxygen saturation. Chest 85:423-428, 1984.

USE OF CONTINUOUS MONITORING OF MIXED VENOUS OXYGEN SATURATION IN THE CORONARY CARE UNIT

5

Joel M. Gore, M.D.*

Dissatisfaction with the thermodilution cardiac output method, coupled with the need for an oximeter to measure pulmonary artery saturation, originally prompted our search for another way of continuously monitoring our patients. We discovered the OXIMETRIX® Opticath® Oximetry System, and it has proven to be highly effective. I will discuss how this System has been used in our coronary care unit (CCU).

*Assistant Professor of Medicine
University of Massachusetts Medical School
Worcester, Massachusetts 01605

The Fick equation, shown in Figure 1, relates that the cardiac output is equal to oxygen consumption divided by the arterial-venous oxygen content difference ($CaO_2 - CvO_2$). When caring for CCU patients, we assume that oxygen consumption stays fairly constant. We can make this assumption because the cardiac patient is on complete bed rest and does not usually have seizures or an elevated temperature. Thus, factors that affect oxygen consumption directly remain fairly constant. Arterial oxygen content also stays fairly constant, in the absence of significant lung disease, because supplemental oxygen is given. Therefore, we can assume that a change in venous oxygen content will be directly related to a change in cardiac output. As venous oxygen content decreases, the $CaO_2 - CvO_2$ increases, representing a decrease in cardiac output.

$$\text{CARDIAC OUTPUT (C.O.)} = \frac{\text{Oxygen consumption (ml/min) X 100}}{\text{Arterial } O_2 \text{ content} - \text{Venous } O_2 \text{ content}}$$

Figure 1

There are many clinical conditions in which the continuous monitoring of mixed venous oxygen saturation ($S\bar{v}O_2$) in a CCU is extremely valuable. The usefulness of the catheter starts while it is being inserted. The diagnostic run is an important and frequently forgotten part of the insertion of a pulmonary artery catheter. Identifying an intracardiac shunt can have a significant impact on the calculation of hemodynamic parameters and the subsequent management of the patient. Patients receiving intra-aortic balloon counterpulsation, in cardiogenic shock with mechanical complications of acute myocardial infarction, or who require hemodynamic monitoring with atrioventricular (AV) sequential pacing, all benefit from continuous monitoring of $S\bar{v}O_2$. Other groups of patients for whom the system is useful include those with cardiac tamponade and those on mechanical ventilation or drug trials.

It must be stressed that it is not a specific measurement or specific number that is important, it is the size and direction of change in the variable being measured that is significant. It does not make any difference if mixed venous O_2 is 70%, 75%, or 76%. What is important is the direction and magnitude of change.

During the routine insertion of a flow-directed pulmonary artery catheter, saturations in each chamber entered should be recorded. This is referred to as the diagnostic run. As shown in Figure 2, saturations are measured in the right atrium (RA), right ventricle (RV), and the pulmonary artery (PA). Normally, there should be very little change in oxygen saturation as one goes through the chambers of the heart.

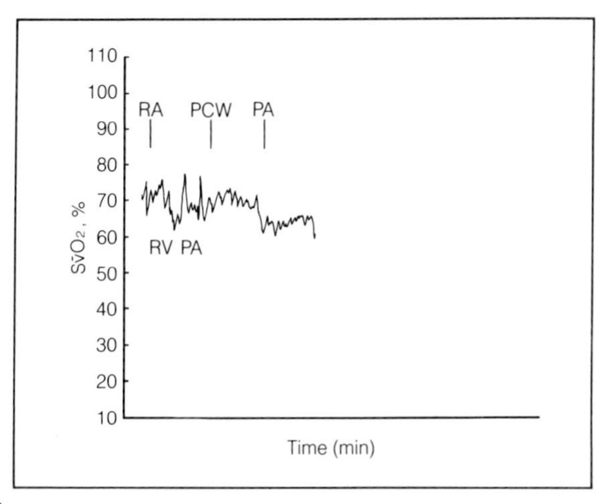

Figure 2
Mixed venuous saturations in the right atrium, right ventricle, and the pulmonary artery recorded during right heart catheterization.

If oxygen saturation or content increases by more than accepted limits, an intracardiac shunt exists at that level. Inflation of the balloon of the catheter to measure pulmonary capillary wedge pressure (PCWP) may impede the fiberoptics and prevent the rise in arterial saturation one would expect of a wedged sample. However, if you do not inflate the balloon and a spontaneous wedge tracing occurs, you will see a dramatic increase in saturation, as shown in Figure 3. For many physicians this is not important; however, when dealing with patients with valvular disease, it is very important to know a confirmed wedge pressure.

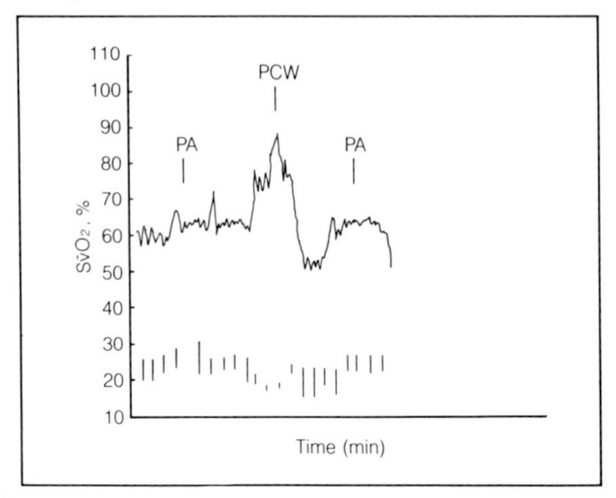

Figure 3
Increased saturation with spontaneous pulmonary capillary wedge.

The performance of the fiberoptic system is reflected in the intensity bars at the bottom of the strip chart recording. It indicates that the fiberoptic system is seeing unimpeded blood flow and that the saturation recorded is fairly accurate. When the catheter is wedged, the intensity bars decrease in length dramatically. We have found that this is a very useful way of determining whether or not the catheter has spontaneously wedged. Frequently, pressure monitoring shows a dampened pressure tracing, and it is necessary to rule out that the catheter has not wedged itself. This is done by using the intensity bars generated by the fiberoptics to determine if the dampened pressure tracing is due to wedging. Short intensity bars usually indicate that catheters are wedged. When adequate intensity bars are present, and there is dampened pressure tracing, it indicates air or blood in the pressure monitoring line.

The importance of the diagnostic run is emphasized in the following case. A 70-year-old patient was transferred to our institution for coronary artery bypass surgery. A physical examination revealed a soft second heart sound and a systolic ejection murmur. He had undergone heart catheterization at the referring hospital, and the calculated aortic valve area was 1.2 cm^2. The calculation of valve area is dependent on cardiac output. In the calculation of this patient's cardiac output a thermodilution output was used that was obtained from right heart catheterization. It was thought that the valve area was noncritical and that only bypass surgery would be needed.

Because of persistent chest pain, an Opticath was inserted preoperatively. The diagnostic run revealed a saturation in the right atrium of 80%. The saturation in the right ventricle was 72%, and in the pulmonary artery 68%. Later, by using green dye, the presence of an atrial septal defect was confirmed. This was a very important finding. In the presence of a left-to-right shunt, thermodilution overestimates the cardiac output. Recalculating the valve area by using the correct cardiac output revealed that the valve area was 0.6 cm^2, an extremely narrowed valve. The patient ended up having aortic valve replacement in addition to bypass surgery and did well. This emphasizes the need to perform diagnostic runs in all patients.

The diagnostic run can also yield extremely important information in the acutely shocky cardiac patient. The patient whose run is shown in Figure 4 presented with an acute myocardial infarction and new holosystolic murmur. On insertion of the Opticath, the saturation in the right atrium was 60%. Entering the right ventricle the saturation rose abruptly to almost 90% and fell back into the 80% range on entering the pulmonary artery. The diagnosis of an acute ventricular septal rupture was made. The patient was managed with an intra-aortic balloon counterpulsation and intravenous nitroprusside, with a resulting drop in his $S\bar{v}O_2$ from 80% to 60%. This was one of the few instances in which a decrease in $S\bar{v}O_2$ actually indicated the patient was getting better. The patient was subsequently taken for cardiac catheterization and surgery where the presence of the rupture was confirmed.

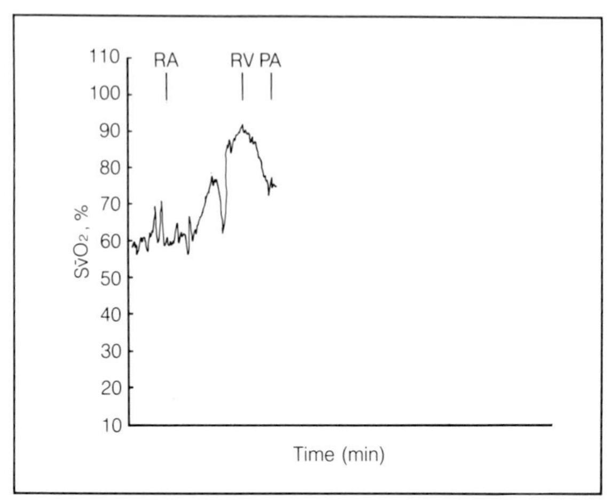

Figure 4
Oxygen saturations in a patient with acute ventricular septal rupture. Note dramatic rise in $S\bar{v}O_2$ as the right ventricle was entered.

Continuous monitoring of $S\bar{v}O_2$ can be helpful when weaning patients from intra-aortic balloon counterpulsation. How do you know when a patient is ready to be weaned? Monitoring $S\bar{v}O_2$ when weaning patients off the balloon can be used to determine whether other therapeutic interventions are needed before removal of the balloon. As shown in Figure 5, changes in $S\bar{v}O_2$ occurred prior to any symptoms or changes in the other hemodynamic parameters that were being monitored.

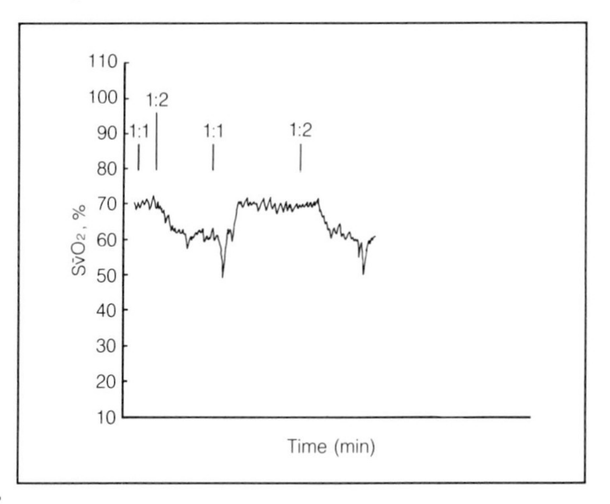

Figure 5
Oxygen saturations during weaning from intra-aortic balloon counterpulsation.

Continuous monitoring of $S\bar{v}O_2$ can be useful in determining prognosis. When $S\bar{v}O_2$ approaches 30% to 40%, significant lactic acidosis is present and prognosis is uniformly poor. We have been able to use this knowledge to give patients and their families some idea of prognosis.

The patient in Figure 6 was in cardiogenic shock with a $S\bar{v}O_2$ of only 35%. An intra-aortic balloon was inserted, and inotropic drugs and vasopressors were started without any improvement. Eighteen hours later, there was a sudden and unexpected increase in $S\bar{v}O_2$. Our initial impression was a miraculous recovery due to our heroic efforts. Somehow we had improved the patient's $S\bar{v}O_2$ and thus the cardiac output, even though we did not know why or how. Two hours later the patient spiked a temperature to 104°F and had a white count of about 50,000/μL. The patient was septic. We did not realize two hours earlier that the increase in $S\bar{v}O_2$ represented sepsis. This patient had a gradual downhill course and died about 24 hours later. In retrospect, this sudden increase in $S\bar{v}O_2$ was our first warning that something was going wrong with the patient.

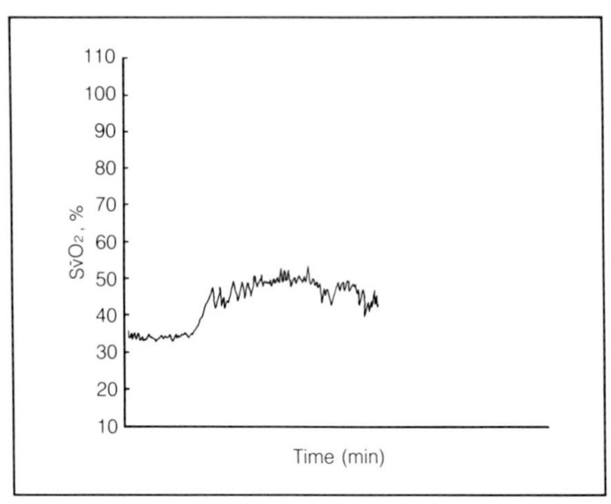

Figure 6

Increase in $S\bar{v}O_2$ prior to onset of symptoms of sepsis in a patient with cardiogenic shock.

A sudden increase in $S\bar{v}O_2$ was seen in another shock patient who initially had an $S\bar{v}O_2$ of 40% to 50% as seen in Figure 7. We were surprised because nothing had really changed with the patient and he was afebrile. What did become apparent several hours later was that the patient had a perforated ulcer that bled into his abdomen. The GI hemorrhage was manifested by a sudden increase in his $S\bar{v}O_2$. Again, the increased $S\bar{v}O_2$ was the earliest warning we had that something was going wrong with the patient.

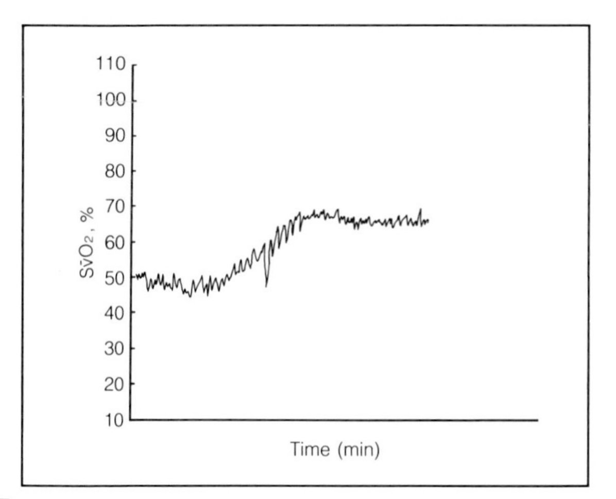

Figure 7
Increase in $S\bar{v}O_2$ associated with GI hemorrhage.

Atrioventricular pacing can improve cardiac output by up to 40% in selected patients. In a patient with an anterior myocardial infarction (MI), AV pacing maintaining normal physiologic conduction through the heart kept the $S\bar{v}O_2$ at 70%. Ventricular pacing at the same heart rate resulted in a 10% to 12% decrease in $S\bar{v}O_2$, and this was reflected in a decrease in thermodilution cardiac output as shown in Figure 8. When we reinstituted AV synchrony, $S\bar{v}O_2$ again increased. In this individual, the synchronized atrial contraction contributed significantly to the cardiac output.

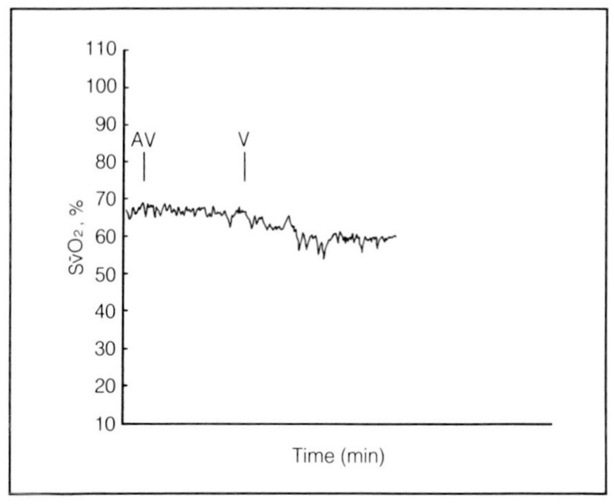

Figure 8
Drop in $S\bar{v}O_2$ associated with change from AV to ventricular pacing in a patient with anterior MI.

Cardiac tamponade is a cardiac emergency requiring immediate intervention. The patient in Figure 9 had all the classic signs of tamponade. On insertion of the catheter, the right atrial pressure was 20 mm Hg, PA pressure was 35/25 mm Hg, and the pericardial pressure was 20 mm Hg. The blood pressure at this time was 110/85 mm Hg. When initially aspirated, the pericardial fluid was bloody. The question that develops is this: What structure are you in? Are you truly in the pericardium, or possibly the right ventricle? In a critically ill patient, a decision is necessary to either proceed or withdraw. In this case, we elected to withdraw 30 to 50 ml of fluid, resulting in a dramatic increase in $S\bar{v}O_2$. The pericardial pressure was 20 mm Hg when we first started, and 20 minutes later it was 19 mm Hg. The right atrial pressure increased to 22 mm Hg, and the PA pressure changed to 35/20 mm Hg. Twenty minutes after starting the pericardiocentesis and removing about 400 ml of fluid, the other hemodynamic parameters (pulse, right atrial pressure, and pericardial pressure) fell. At this point, we felt comfortable that we had therapeutically treated this patient. Again, the earliest indication we had that what we were doing was therapeutically beneficial to the patient was obtained by continuously monitoring $S\bar{v}O_2$.

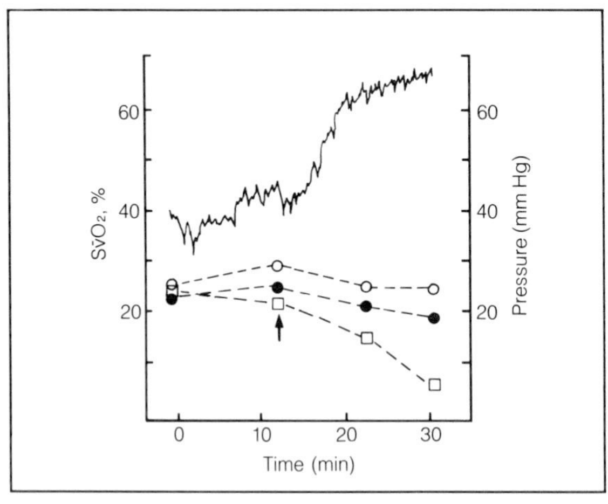

Figure 9

Change in pulmonary arterial $S\bar{v}O_2$ over time. Time 0 corresponds to time when pericardiocentesis was started. Twelve minutes later (arrow), after verification of catheter position in pressure measurements, fluid was removed. Improvement in pulmonary arterial $S\bar{v}O_2$ over the next ten minutes corresponds to removal of 300 ml of fluid. Also plotted are mean right atrial pressure (●), mean pulmonary arterial pressure (○), and mean pericardial pressure (□).

A sudden unexpected drop in $S\bar{v}O_2$ should prompt a search for the change in cardiac status. Critically ill individuals are frequently dependent on pharmacologic agents. As shown in Figure 10, the sudden drop in $S\bar{v}O_2$ prompted a search for the cause. The dobutamine was discovered to be infusing into the bed, rather than into the patient. Reinstituting dobutamine therapy resulted in a return to baseline. Again, the earliest sign we had that something had gone wrong was a change in $S\bar{v}O_2$.

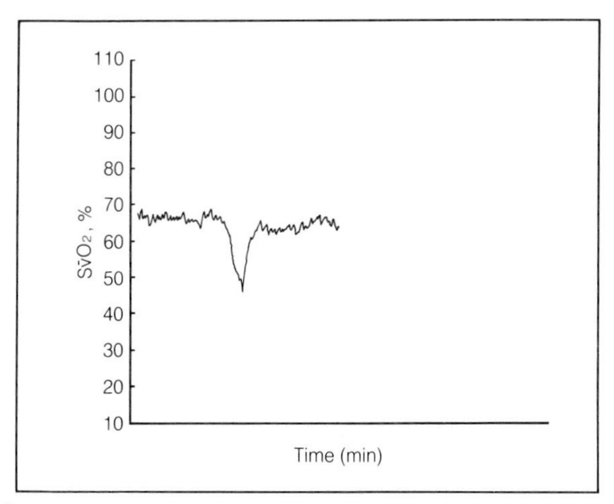

Figure 10
Fall in $S\bar{v}O_2$ occuring with disconnection of dobutamine infusion.

Continuous monitoring of $S\bar{v}O_2$ has proven very helpful in our work with a new investigational inotropic agent. To assess the effectiveness of this new agent, all patients must undergo measurement of right heart hemodynamic variables. The effectiveness of this new agent can be seen by following cardiac output and $S\bar{v}O_2$. As shown in Figure 11, baseline cardiac output was 4.2 L/min and $S\bar{v}O_2$ was 57%. Five minutes after the drug was given, the $S\bar{v}O_2$ rose to 67%. After 15 minutes, the saturation went up to 68%. At two hours, after the drug had worn off, hemodynamically the patient returned to baseline with an $S\bar{v}O_2$ of 60%. A larger dose of the drug was then given. Five minutes after giving the drug, the $S\bar{v}O_2$ went up to 73% and peaked at 76%. Two hours later, it fell back down to baseline. If, after administering a drug, you can assess the effectiveness by monitoring $S\bar{v}O_2$, it is much simpler than following cardiac outputs.

THE EFFECTS OF AN INVESTIGATIONAL INOTROPIC AGENT ON MIXED VENOUS OXYGEN SATURATION

Patient 1	H.R.	$\overline{RAP}$	$\overline{PAP}$	PAP	PCWP	CO	$S\bar{v}O_2$
Baseline	78	4	56/22	34	20	4.2	57
1 mg + 5 min	80	6	58/25	35	23	N.P.	67
1 mg + 15 min	81	5	51/23	32	18	4.7	68
1 mg + 2 hr	95	4	69/31	46	24	3.6	60
2 mg + 5 min	103	0	58/25	38	22	6.9	73
2 mg + 15 min	97	0	40/15	25	10	6.2	76
2 mg + 2 hr	94	1	66/33	40	21	4.5	62
Patient 2							
Baseline	65	31	57/30	39	30	2.4	40
1 mg + 5 min	80	23	56/27	50	27	4.8	51
1 mg + 15 min	60	25	64/27	38	27	2.8	44
1 mg + 2 hr	66	28	56/30	39	30	2.5	42
2 mg + 5 min	84	19	52/25	35	22	4.8	68
2 mg + 15 min	66	19	55/20	33	23	4.4	58
2 mg + 2 hr	74	20	60/27	37	27	3.4	48

Key

H.R.–heart rate
$\overline{RAP}$–mean right atrial pressure
$\overline{PAP}$–mean pulmonary artery pressure
PAP–pulmonary artery pressure
PCWP–pulmonary capillary wedge pressure
CO–cardiac output
$S\bar{v}O_2$–mixed venous oxygen saturation
N.P.–not performed

Figure 11

In conclusion, I would like to share with you what we have found to be the advantages of continuously measuring $S\bar{v}O_2$ in the CCU as listed in Figure 12. We have found that it gives us the earliest identification of hemodynamic and clinical changes in patients. We have not found anything that identifies these changes any earlier. It helps us to optimize patient management by the immediate assessment of the efficacy of our intervention, be it pericardiocentesis or the institution of a new inotropic agent. There is a decrease in cost since multiple blood samples are not required for oximetry analysis. Finally, there is decreased work for medical and paramedical personnel since one instrument supplies multiple pieces of information on the patient. This early warning system for both diagnostic and therapeutic intervention analysis has improved our ability to care for selected critically ill patients.

ADVANTAGES OF CONTINUOUS MONITORING OF MIXED VENOUS OXYGEN SATURATION

1. Early identification of hemodynamic and clinical changes in patients.
2. Optimization of patient management by immediate assessment of the efficacy of an intervention.
3. Decreased cost since multiple blood samples are not required for oximetry analysis.
4. Decreased work for medical and paramedical personnel since one instrument supplies multiple pieces of information.

Figure 12

THE OXIMETRIX® OPTICATH® OXIMETRY SYSTEM: THEORY AND DEVELOPMENT

6

John M. Sperinde, Ph.D.*
Kathi M. Senelly, B.S.*

Oximeters designed to measure oxygen saturation *in vivo* were first used more than 25 years ago in an attempt to eliminate the need for repeated blood sampling and to obtain oxygen saturation information in a more timely manner. More recently, OXIMETRIX developed improved technology for continuous *in vivo* measurement of blood oxygen saturation and produced a reliable, practical, and accurate catheter oximetry system.

*OXIMETRIX, Inc.
1212 Terra Bella Avenue
Mountain View, California 94043

PRINCIPLES OF SPECTROPHOTOMETRIC BLOOD OXYGEN MEASUREMENT

Standard laboratory measurement technique for determining blood oxygen saturation utilizes spectrophotometry to differentiate oxygenated blood from deoxygenated blood. Light of selected wavelengths is transmitted through a cuvette containing a blood sample, as illustrated in Figure 1. Wavelengths are chosen so that the absorption characteristics of oxyhemoglobin and hemoglobin are different as in Figure 2. The light transmitted through the sample at each wavelength varies, depending on the relative concentrations of oxyhemoglobin and hemoglobin. Thus, by analyzing the light transmitted through the sample at different wavelengths, the ratio of hemoglobin to oxyhemoglobin can be determined.[1]

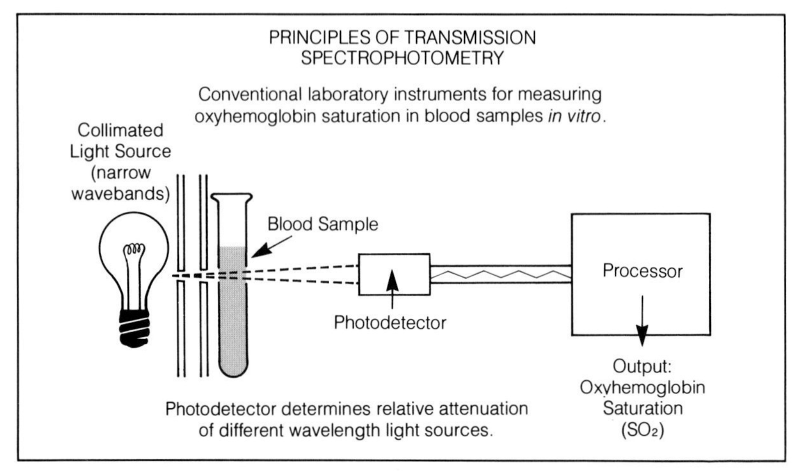

Figure 1

Transmission spectrophotometry involves transmission of light of selected wavelengths through a blood sample and analysis of the light transmitted through the sample to determine the ratio of hemoglobin to oxyhemoglobin.

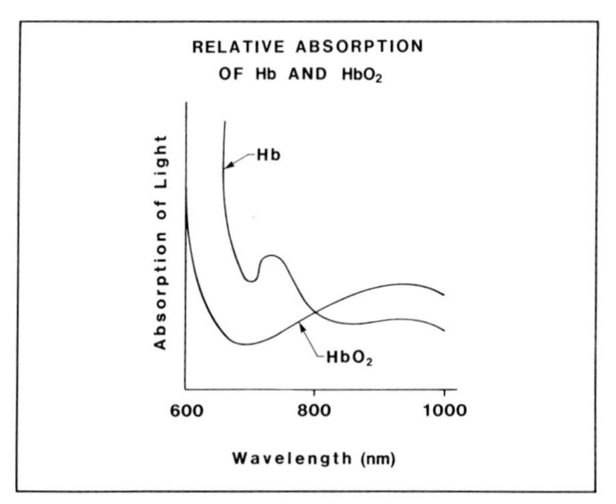

Figure 2
The absorption characteristics of hemoglobin (Hb) and oxyhemoglobin (HbO_2) are a function of the wavelengths of the light being transmitted through the sample.

This same principle is used in *in vivo* oximetry instruments, which use reflection spectrophotometry rather than the transmission method. The principles of measurement are the same, except that the light that is analyzed is backscattered or reflected and refracted by the blood cells. This is shown in Figures 3 and 4.[2,3] This allows the light source and the detector to be on the same side of the blood sample and therefore eliminates the need for the sample to be placed in a cuvette.[2]

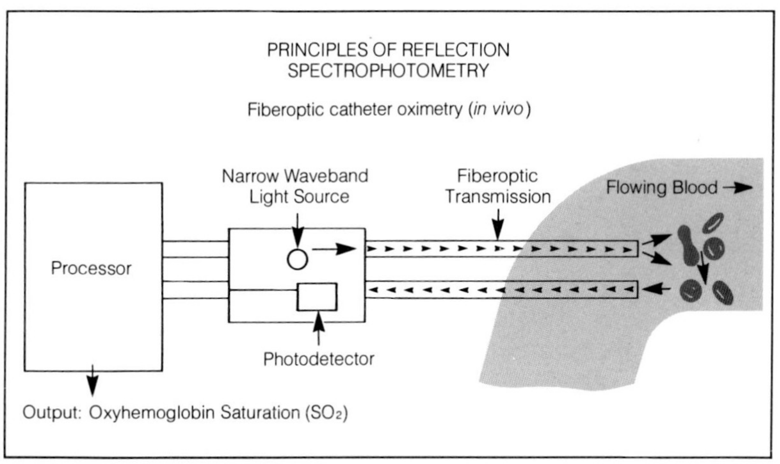

Figure 3
Reflection spectrophotometry requires the measurement of light reflected (backscattered) by blood cells.

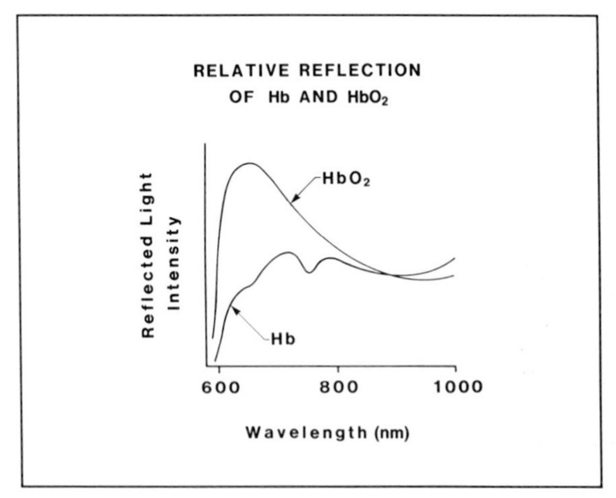

Figure 4

In the same manner as absorption, reflection characteristics of hemoglobin and oxyhemoglobin are a function of wavelength. For example, when light at a wavelength of approximately 660 nm is used, oxyhemoglobin reflects much more light than hemoglobin.

HISTORICAL PERSPECTIVE: *IN VIVO* OXIMETRY TECHNOLOGY

Fiberoptic *in vivo* reflection oximeters have been used for approximately 25 years.[4] In the past, two wavelengths were used for oxygen saturation measurement. Usually one of these wavelengths was 805 nm, which is the wavelength at which oxyhemoglobin and hemoglobin absorb light equally; the other selected wavelength was typically about 660 nm, the wavelength at which the difference in light absorption characteristics between hemoglobin and oxyhemoglobin is maximized.[5,6] Pairs of light pulses at these two wavelengths were sent through a fiberoptic bundle to illuminate flowing blood. The amount of reflected light of each wavelength was detected and a ratio was computed.

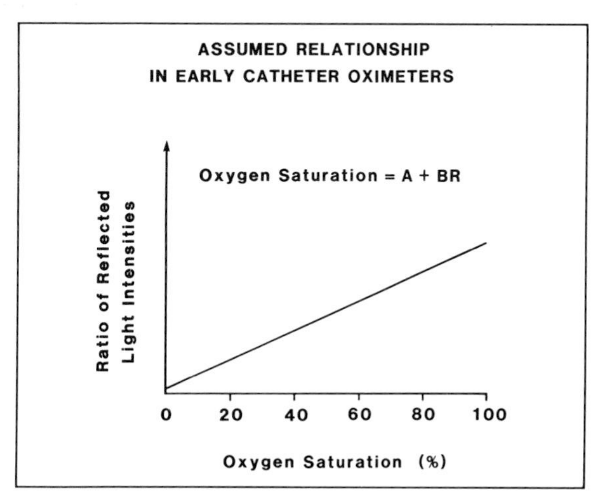

Figure 5
Early in vivo *oximeters operated on the assumption that the oxygen saturation was a linear function of the ratio of reflected light at two selected wavelengths.*

The Assumed Correlation Relationship

With early *in vivo* oximeters, oxygen saturation was assumed to be a linear function of the reflected light ratio as illustrated in Figure 5. It was calculated from an equation of the following form:

$$\text{Oxygen Saturation} = A + BR$$

where A was a constant that varied from one bundle of fiberoptics to another, B was a constant determined from analysis of a blood sample, and R was the ratio of light intensities.[7]

This assumption (that oxygen saturation was a linear function of the light ratio) was a serious problem with these early oximeters. In reality, oxygen saturation is not a linear function of the light intensity ratio. Further, various routinely occurring changes in the blood (pH, hematocrit, and blood flow velocity changes, for instance) affect the apparent color of blood and therefore also affect this relationship.[3] As shown in Figure 6, the nonlinearities and changes associated with these various factors meant that there was a range of oxygen saturation values that would result in the same reflected light intensity ratio. An oxygen saturation value could be calculated by assuming a linear relationship, but the value would not necessarily be sufficiently accurate or reliable to be useful in routine clinical application.

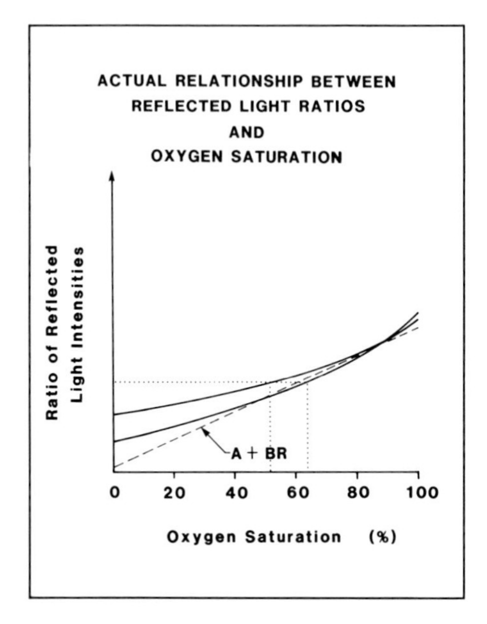

Figure 6

The relationship between the reflected light ratio and oxygen saturation is represented by these curves, where changes in hematocrit, pH, blood flow velocity, and other physiological factors can alter the relationship within this "envelope." Thus, any given light ratio could represent a relatively broad range of oxygen saturations (as indicated by the dotted lines).

Calibration

A second major drawback that prevented widespread acceptance of these early *in vivo* oximeters had to do with calibration of the systems; that is, the determination of the A and B constants (the slope and intercept) of the assumed linear correlation relationship. Some of the early systems required a two-point calibration involving immersion of the catheter tip in blood samples with two different known oxygen saturations. This provided the information necessary to determine the slope and intercept of the linear equation used to calculate oxygen saturation from *in vivo* measurements.[7] This two-point calibration was required due to the optical limitations inherent in the design and construction of the catheters.

The catheters were typically constructed with bundles consisting of multiple fiberoptic filaments. Arrangement of the numerous sending and receiving fibers at the tip of the catheter was either uncontrolled (in an attempt to have a random pattern), or in a definite pattern, as exemplified in Figure 7a. The key parameter affecting the calibration constants for a particular catheter was the average optical distance between sending and receiving fiberoptics.[8,9]

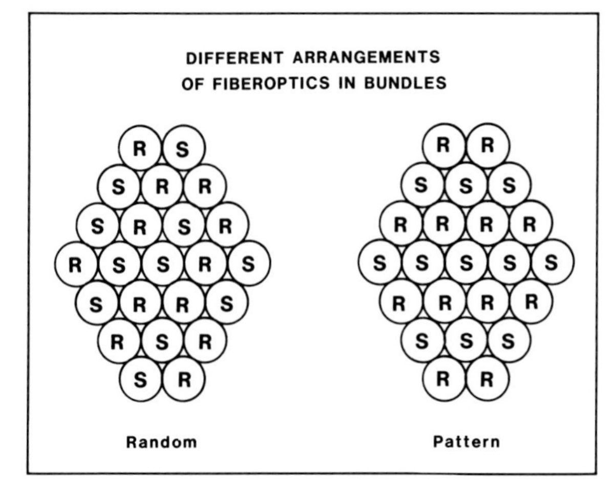

Figure 7a

Bundles of fiberoptics are either randomly arranged (as on the left) or arranged in a specific pattern (shown on the right). The sending fibers are labeled with an "S," and receiving fibers are labeled with an "R."

For the random array, an assumption was typically made that the average of the distances between the various sending and receiving fiberoptics would be the same for all catheters. Unfortunately, the numbers of fibers in an individual catheter and the random nature of the fiber mixing was never sufficient to achieve a fixed average distance, and thus unique calibration for each catheter was necessary.

The patterned array was an attempt to overcome the inability to obtain a true random pattern with a limited number of fibers. Even in this case it was not possible to achieve uniform average optical distance between sending and receiving fiberoptics. For example, consider a simple case as in Figure 7b, in which all the sending fibers and all the receiving fibers are in separate but adjacent rows. In this case, S_1-R_1, S_2-R_2, S_3-R_3, and S_4-R_4 are uniformly spaced with respect to each other. However, this distance is different from the distance between S_1 and R_3, S_2 and R_4, and so on. In addition, differences in light transmission characteristics between individual fibers (due to a lack of uniformity in producing the fibers or as a result of damage or breakage) would completely change the optical pattern and, therefore, the calibration.[8,9]

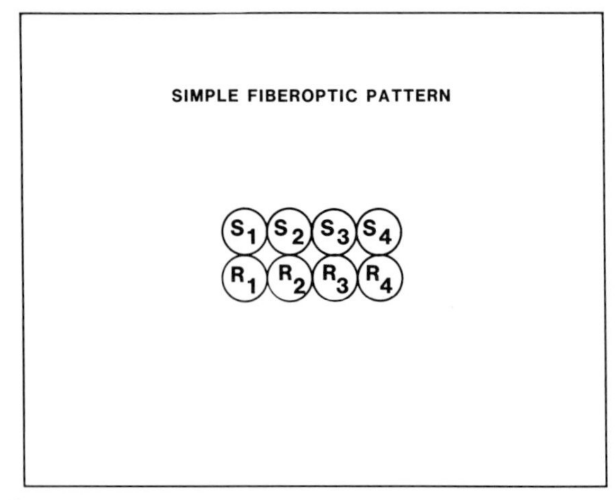

Figure 7b

With sending and receiving fibers in separate rows, some distances between fibers are uniform (S_1 to R_1, S_2 to R_2, etc.) but are not equal to other distances (the distance between S_1 and R_3 is not equal to the distance between S_1 and R_1).

The inconvenience of the two-point method of calibration could be slightly reduced if the catheter manufacturer provided one of the linear equation constants. Generally, the constant provided was the intercept A, which, because it was a function of the optical geometry at the catheter tip, was unique to each catheter. With this constant provided, only one blood sample measurement was necessary to determine the other constant and thus fully define the assumed linear equation.[7]

An alternative method of calibration involved the use of sterile milk of magnesia as a reflection standard. The catheter tip was inserted into the reflection medium, and intensity of light reflected at the two wavelengths was set at equality, but this could not compensate for the geometric variations described previously. The tip was then rinsed before insertion into the patient.[10,11]

Vessel Wall Artifact

A third serious shortcoming of the early oximeters was related to their inability to compensate adequately for large fluctuations in the reflected light signal due to periodic vessel wall artifact. This vessel wall artifact is usually related to the cardiac and respiratory cycles since it is a function of the motion of the catheter tip relative to the blood vessel walls.[7]

The light intensity changes significantly even within a single cardiac cycle as shown in Figure 8. The high peaks in the reflected light

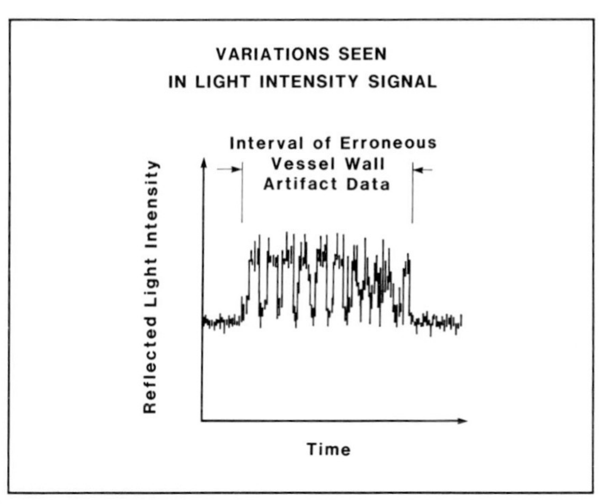

Figure 8

The light intensity signal varies significantly as a result of vessel wall artifact due to catheter tip movement during the cardiac and respiratory cycles.

intensity represent light being reflected from vessel walls rather than from the blood. The spectral characteristic of light reflected from a blood vessel wall is typically similar to that reflected from blood in the 85% to 95% saturation range. Using such signals without filtering out the vessel wall artifact thus produced readings that were very erratic and falsely elevated like the example in Figure 9a. In order to get a clinically usable tracing, the signals could be averaged over a long period of time and presented as a "smoothed" stable value. However, the value so determined for the oxygen saturation would be at a different level than the actual oxygen saturation due to the inclusion of the wall signals in the average. This can be seen in Figure 9b.[12]

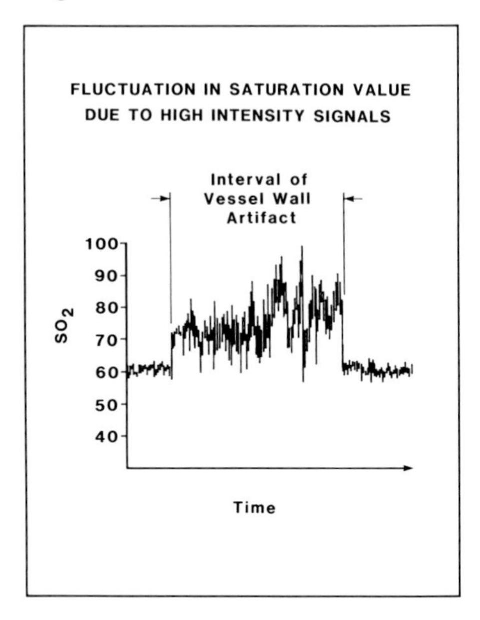

Figure 9a
This tracing represents periods of high intensity vessel wall artifact, as seen if the light signals are not filtered.

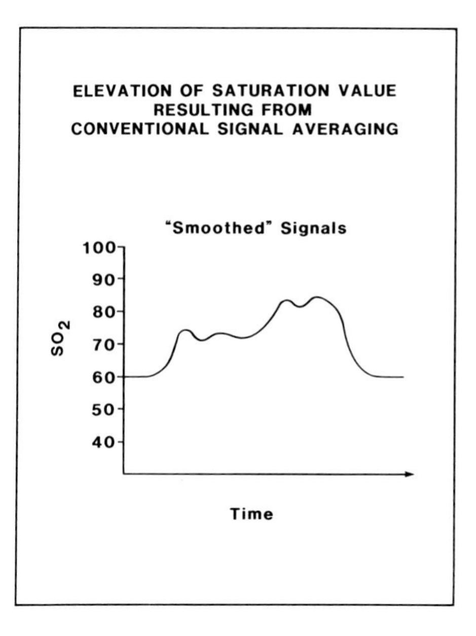

Figure 9b
Simply averaging the signal over long periods of time will result in a "smooth" curve that has been falsely elevated by the vessel wall artifact.

Catheter Stiffness

A fourth major problem with early catheter oximeters was related to the stiffness and fragility of fiberoptic catheters, which made them impractical or unacceptable for routine clinical use. The early *in vivo* oximeters used bundles of glass fiberoptics that were inserted into arterial needles, double-lumen cardiac catheters, or triple-lumen pulmonary artery catheters.[13] When plastic optical fibers became available, they were used in the bundles instead of glass fibers in order to reduce the possibility of fiber breakage.[7]

OXIMETRIX OPTICATH OXIMETRY SYSTEM DESIGN

The OXIMETRIX Opticath Oximetry System consists of an electronic Processor, several types of arterial and pulmonary artery catheters, an optical reference standard packaged with each catheter, and an Optical Module. The System is designed to continuously monitor oxygen saturation in an accurate, reliable, and safe manner. These System components are illustrated in Figures 10 and 11.

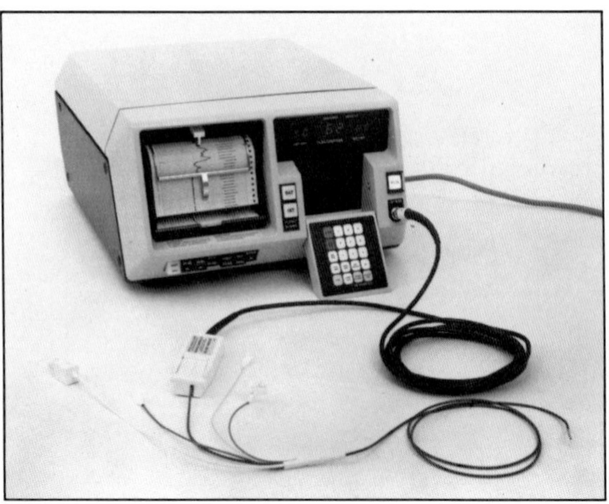

Figure 10
The Model 1270A OXIMETRIX Opticath Oximetry System.

Processor

The Processor, or Oximetry Instrument, is a microprocessor-controlled device that performs sophisticated digital processing of electrical signals. The Model 1270A Processor provides a numerical readout of oxygen saturation, a continuous chart recording of oxygen saturation, and an "intensity" measurement that provides the clinician with an indication of the quality of optical signals being received. These features have been shown to be clinically useful in patient monitoring; the digital display of saturation provides continuously updated information on the current oxygen saturation, and the chart recording allows the patient's oxygen saturation history to be easily reviewed.[14] In addition, the display of reflected light intensity allows quick detection of changes in catheter position, fiberoptics integrity, and adequacy of signal. Audible and visual alarms alert the user to changes in oxygen saturation and signal intensity.

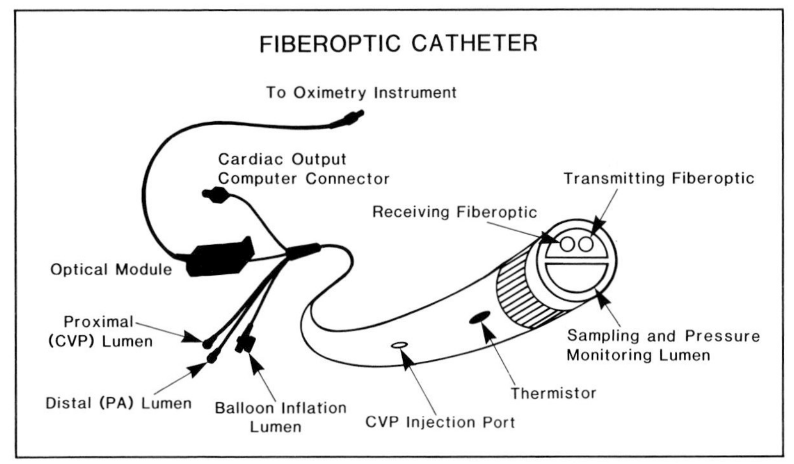

Figure 11

The catheter used with the OXIMETRIX Opticath Oximetry System transmits light to the blood through one optical fiber and returns the reflected light through a second optical fiber. The catheter is optically connected to the Oximetry Processor through the Optical Module.

The necessary accuracy of the OXIMETRIX Opticath Oximetry System has been achieved through the development of techniques that allow three wavelengths, rather than two as in older systems, to be used for oxygen saturation measurement. Using patent-protected techniques, the Oximetry System uses three carefully selected wavelengths that allow two independent light ratios to be determined, as illustrated in Figure 12, rather than one such ratio as in two wavelength instruments. An appropriate combination of these two independent ratios of light intensities reduces the instrument's sensitivity to physiological factors such as hematocrit and pulsatile flow, as well as changes in light scattering from red blood cell surfaces and blood vessel walls.[15,16]

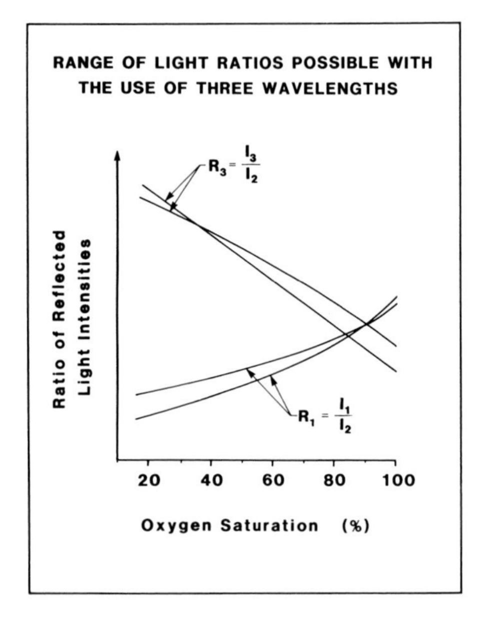

Figure 12

The use of three wavelengths of light allows two light ratios to be computed and used for determination of oxygen saturation.

With the OXIMETRIX System, carboxyhemoglobin is detected as an almost nonabsorbing substance and therefore does not significantly affect the oxygen saturation value. This can been seen in Figure 13, in which the absorption spectrum for carboxyhemoglobin is shown with the spectra for hemoglobin and oxyhemoglobin.[1,17] In effect, the absorption of carboxyhemoglobin (HbCO) is roughly one-fourteenth that of hemoglobin. In other words, a 14% carboxyhemoglobin level would reduce the computed saturation by approximately 1%. (For additional information, refer to the Supplement at the end of this chapter.)

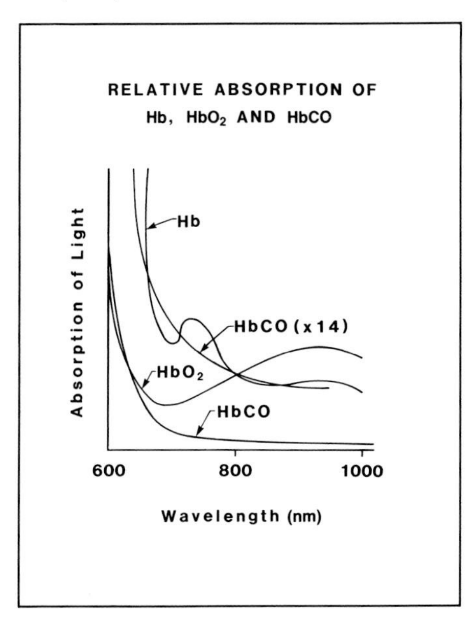

Figure 13

The absorption of carboxyhemoglobin is only one-fourteenth that of reduced hemoglobin, as shown in this comparison of absorption spectra. For comparison purposes, the carboxyhemoglobin spectrum is shown to scale and also amplified by a factor of 14.

As previously discussed, a limitation of early oximeters was their inability to differentiate the frequently occurring vessel wall artifacts from blood signals. Using a patented digital signal filtering technique, the OXIMETRIX instrument continuously analyzes the raw optical data and is able to filter out "noise" coming from vessel wall reflections from data that comes from the blood "signals" as shown in Figure 14.[12] Clinical experience has shown that fiberoptic catheters in critically ill patients may detect noise that is five times the size of the blood signal; the OXIMETRIX digital filter is able to extract the true signal (reflected by the blood) in such cases.

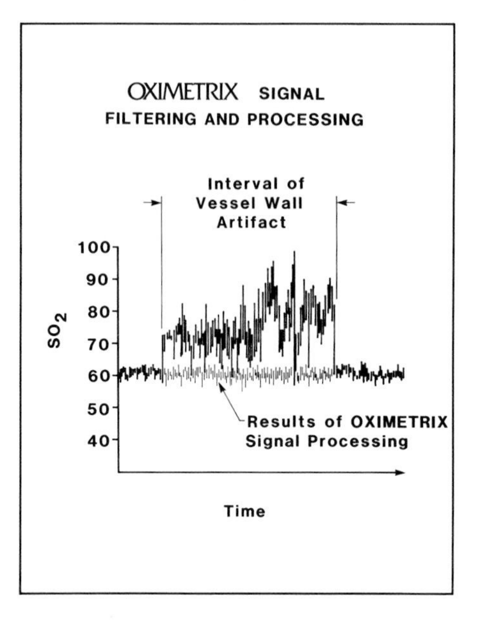

Figure 14
The sophisticated processing performed by the OXIMETRIX Opticath Oximetry System eliminates false elevation of oxygen saturation measurements by detecting and discarding artifact data.

Optical Module

The Optical Module is the optical and electrical interface between the catheter and the Processor. It contains three light-emitting diodes that illuminate, via one of the optical fibers in the catheter, the blood flowing past the catheter tip. The Optical Module also contains a photodetector that receives reflected light returned through a second optical fiber and converts the light intensity levels into electrical signals. These signals are transmitted to the Processor for analysis and processing.

Catheters

Several types of fiberoptic catheters are available for use with the Processor. The most frequently used catheter is the Model P7110. This is a 7.5 French fiberoptic flow-directed thermodilution pulmonary artery catheter, which has been shown to be similar in flexibility and handling characteristics to the nonfiberoptic 7 French catheters made by other manufacturers.[18] Without compromising the ability to withstand longitudinal forces on the catheter, this flexibility has been achieved by threading the catheter with aramid fibers as stress relief for the optical fibers, thereby eliminating the need for unusually stiff catheter material. In addition, elimination of this stiff material allows bending of the catheter to a radius as small as 0.25 in without damaging the fiberoptics.

Calibration and Standardization

Two types of calibration techniques have been incorporated into the OXIMETRIX Opticath Oximetry System. The most accurate form of calibration is actually a standardization of the catheter prior to insertion into the patient. By using single, monofilament optical fibers for each of the transmitting and receiving fibers and closely controlling their optical spacing in all catheters by using a patent-protected method and design, OXIMETRIX has been able to achieve an optical design with sufficient consistency from catheter to catheter to permit this type of universal calibration.[9] Even changes in transmission, while affecting the magnitude of the light intensity signal, do not affect the optical measuring geometry and therefore do not change this calibration.

The standardization technique used in the OXIMETRIX System involves an optical reference that is included in each catheter package. Use of the patent-protected optical reference allows calibration against an absolute color standard, rather than against a blood sample and blood sample measurement, as in Figure 15.[19] This eliminates variability associated with blood samples that are not representative of normal blood. It also avoids a variety of errors associated with the measured value of a sample, including sample handling techniques, calibration of the *in vitro* sample device, and (if saturation is calculated from blood gases rather than actually measured with a laboratory oximeter) the well-known errors associated with calculated saturation values.[20, 21, 22, 23]

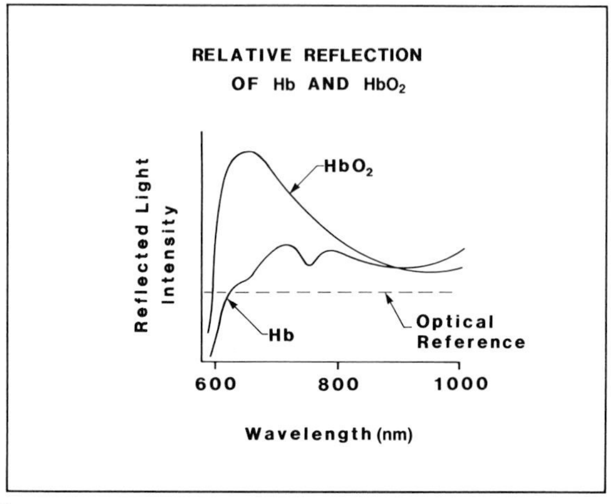

Figure 15

For system calibration, the optical reference provides a color standard that is a known and absolute value rather than a value representative of a particular saturation.

Thus, calibration is *not* performed against a "known" saturation. It is performed against a precisely controlled color reference, and all spectrophotometric measurements made during operation are compared to this reference. Furthermore, standardization in the catheter package provides a check of the OXIMETRIX Opticath Oximetry System prior to use and readies the catheter so that oxygen saturation values obtained at different points during catheter insertion can be used for diagnostic purposes. This OXIMETRIX technological breakthrough simplifies the clinical process of setting up the instrument to obtain accurate readings while improving accuracy by eliminating the dependence upon blood sampling values.

In addition to standardization in the catheter package, an *in vivo* calibration may also be performed if the need arises. This should be done if the catheter is inserted without using the optical reference for standardization, if the fiberoptics are significantly damaged, or if the catheter has been left in place for a considerable length of time. An *in vivo* calibration may be accurate at the time it is performed; however, the oxygen saturation values may not remain accurate with changes in saturation values or other blood parameters such as pH or hematocrit. Figure 6 illustrates the range of intensity ratios that can represent a particular oxygen saturation value. When performing an *in vivo* calibration, the system must make the assumption that the oxygen saturation lies on a curve in the middle of this range. If the blood color is affected by physiological factors, the oxygen saturation may, however, actually lie on a different curve. For this reason, standardizing the catheter against the known color reference provided with the catheter will provide a more accurate and reliable measurement than an *in vivo* calibration.

In practice, of course, the accuracy of *in vivo* calibration can be further compromised by blood sampling measurement errors. Such errors may result from one or more of a variety of factors such as poor sampling technique (that is, if air was allowed into the sample or if the sample was taken when the patient was not clinically stable),[20, 21] computation of oxygen saturation from blood gases rather than actual measurement,[22, 23] inclusion by the laboratory instrument of carboxyhemoglobin in the total hemoglobin amount (refer to the Supplement for additional information), or improper calibration of the laboratory instrument.[21]

SUMMARY

The value of continuous monitoring of oxygen saturation in critically ill patients has been recognized for many years. However, the development of a reliable, simple, and accurate instrument for this monitoring is relatively recent.

With any type of patient monitoring equipment, accuracy and reliability are essential. Through years of clinical and engineering research, OXIMETRIX has developed signal processing algorithms that allow blood signals to be analyzed without incorporating information from erroneous artifact signals. Use of three wavelengths of light, rather than two, for oxygen saturation measurement eliminates some of the sources of error that plagued earlier *in vivo* fiberoptic oximeters.

Simplicity is another important factor to be considered with any instrument used in hospitals. Calibration is easily performed through the use of one of two types of calibration techniques incorporated into the OXIMETRIX Opticath Oximetry System. In most cases, use of the fiberoptic catheters presents no unusual problems because the Model P7110 Opticath catheter is similar in function and handling characteristics to other pulmonary artery flotation catheters.

The OXIMETRIX Opticath Oximetry System has been designed to be a system that accurately and reliably measures oxygen saturation continuously and is practical and easy to use in the clinical environment. Its advent has provided the clinician with a means to continuously measure an important parameter in managing the clinical course of the critically ill patient.

SUPPLEMENT

The OXIMETRIX Opticath Oximetry System defines and computes oxygen saturation according to the following formula:

$$SO_2 = \frac{HbO_2}{Hb + HbO_2} \times 100\%$$

where SO_2 is oxygen saturation, Hb is hemoglobin, and HbO_2 is oxyhemoglobin.

Under normal circumstances, carboxyhemoglobin and methemoglobin do not affect the oxygen saturation measurement since they are not considered in the total amount of hemoglobin. Since these two forms of hemoglobin do not have oxygen-carrying capabilities, the value shown by the OXIMETRIX Opticath Oximetry System reflects the amount of usable hemoglobin that is bound with oxygen.

In cases of carbon monoxide poisoning, the presence of carboxyhemoglobin in excess of 14% of the total hemoglobin content can affect the percentage oxygen saturation calculated from this equation, by being detected as hemoglobin. However, a 14% carboxyhemoglobin level would cause only a 1% reduction in the oxygen saturation value.

Some laboratory oximeters define and compute oxygen saturation with the following equation:

$$SO_2 = \frac{HbO_2}{Hb + HbO_2 + HbCO + HbMet} \times 100\%$$

where HbCO is carboxyhemoglobin, and HbMet is methemoglobin.

Similarly, the other substances can be written as a percentage of the total hemoglobin amount. For example, the percent carboxyhemoglobin would be as follows:

$$\%HbCO = \frac{HbCO}{Hb + HbO_2 + HbCO + HbMet} \times 100\%$$

When determining the oxygen saturation of a blood sample, the value computed by the OXIMETRIX Opticath Oximetry System will always be slightly higher than that determined by a laboratory oximeter using this equation. This stems from the inclusion of carboxyhemoglobin and methemoglobin in the total hemoglobin amount. This difference is especially noticeable in carbon monoxide poisoning, when carboxyhemoglobin can become a significant amount of the total hemoglobin without affecting the System saturation reading. If desired, the laboratory oximeter measurement can be adjusted to reflect the type of value displayed by the System. This entails subtracting the amount of carboxyhemoglobin and methemoglobin from the total hemoglobin amount, and recalculating the oxygen saturation. Thus, the OXIMETRIX Opticath Oximetry System measurement can be correlated with such a laboratory oximeter by using the following equation:

$$SO_2\ (OXIMETRIX) = \frac{SO_2\ (Lab)}{1 - \frac{\%HbCO + \%HbMet}{100}}$$

REFERENCES

1. Glasser, O., editor: Medical Physics, Volume II. Year Book Publishers, Chicago, Illinois:1039-1089, 1950.
2. Zijlstra, W. G. and Mook, G. A.: Medical Reflection Photometry. Royal Van Gorcum Ltd., Assen, The Netherlands, 1962.
3. Mook, G. A., et al: Fibre optic reflection photometry on blood. Cardiovasc. Res. 2:199-209, 1968.
4. Polanyi, M. L. and Hehir, R. M.: *In vivo* oximeter with fast dynamic response. Rev. Sci. Instrum. 33:1050-1054, 1962.
5. Enson, Y., et al: *In vivo* studies with an intravascular and intracardiac reflection oximeter. J. Appl. Physiol. 17:552-558, 1962.
6. Kapany, N. S. and Silbertrust, N.: Fibre optics spectrophotometer for *in vivo* oximetry. Nature 204:138-142, 1964.
7. Martin, W. E., et al: Continuous monitoring of mixed venous oxygen saturation in man. Anesth. Analg. 52:784-793, 1973.
8. Shaw, R. F. and Sperinde, J. M.: U.S. Patent 4,295,470, 1981.
9. Shaw, R. F. and Sperinde, J. M.: U.S. Patent 4,416,285, 1983.
10. Frommer, P. L., et al: Clinical applications of an improved, rapidly responding fiberoptic catheter. Am. J. Cardiol. 15:672-679, 1965.
11. Gamble, W. J., et al: The use of fiberoptics in clinical cardiac catheterization. I. Intracardiac oximetry. Circulation 31:328-343, 1965.
12. Sperinde, J. M., Goldring, S. D., Miller, D. T.: U.S. Patent 4,453,218, 1984.
13.. Kapany, N. S., et al: Fiber optics oximeter-densitometer for cardiovascular studies. Applied Optics 6:565-570, 1967.
14. Baele, P.L., et al: Continuous monitoring of mixed venous oxygen saturation in critically ill patients. Anesth. Analg. 61:513-517, 1982.
15. Shaw, R. F.: U.S. Patent 3,638,640, 1972.
16. Shaw, R. F. and Sperinde, J. M.: U.S. Patent 4,114,604, 1978.
17. Gordy, E. and Drabkin, D. L.: Spectrophotometric Studies XVI. Determination of the oxygen saturation of blood by a simplified technique, applicable to standard equipment. J. Biol. Chem. 227:285-299, 1957.
18. McMichan, J. C., Baele, P. L. and Wignes, M. W.: Insertion of pulmonary artery catheters — a comparison of fiberoptic and nonfiberoptic catheters. Crit. Care Med. 12:517-519, 1984.
19. Shaw, R. F. and Sperinde, J. M.: U.S. Patent 4,322,164, 1982.
20. Brantigan, J. W.: Accuracy of clinical blood gas measurements (letter to the editor). JAMA 229:1723, 1974.
21. Shrout, J. B.: Controlling the quality of blood gas results. Am. J. Med. Tech. 48:347-351, 1982.
22. Thomas, L. J.: Algorithms for selected blood acid-base and blood gas calculations. J. Appl. Physiol. 33:154-158, 1972.
23. Riley, J. B. and Palmer-Steele, C.L.: Hemoglobin P_{50} dynamics during hypothermic cardiopulmonary bypass. J.E.C.T. 15:167-170, 1983.

IS CONTINUOUS MEASUREMENT OF BLOOD OXYGEN SATURATION A SIGNIFICANT ADVANCE IN HEMODYNAMIC MONITORING AND MANAGEMENT OF THE HIGH RISK PATIENT?

7

PANEL DISCUSSION
QUESTIONS AND ANSWERS

Arnold Aberman, M.D., F.A.C.P.
Patrick J. Fahey, M.D.
Joel M. Gore, M.D.
John C. McMichan, M.B., B.S., Ph.D.
Paul M. Stevens, M.D.

QUESTION: Dr. McMichan showed a slide that indicated synchronous intermittent mandatory ventilation (SIMV) was effective in ventilating a patient, while Dr. Fahey showed the reverse. Can you explain?

MCMICHAN: We are looking at two different patients at two different times, and they are not comparable. In some patients one particular mode of ventilation is appropriate for that patient at that particular time. A lot of us up to now have used educated clinical guesses to decide what mode of ventilation is appropriate for that patient at that time. We now have a means of either supporting or disagreeing with our educated clinical guesses: We can watch the response as we change the mode. Dr. Fahey's patient did not like it, and mine happened to like it. I have patients like his that did not like it, and I am sure he has the reverse. It is the patient at the time.

QUESTION: What magnitude of decrease in mixed venous oxygen saturation ($S\bar{v}O_2$) is significant in a patient with a stable baseline?

FAHEY: That is an important question. Clinically, I am not certain we have the answer yet. We are still using this as a primary monitoring device. As Dr. Aberman mentioned, when we first had around-the-clock ECG monitoring, we could see two or three premature ventricular contractions (PVCs) and maybe not think much about it. When we had more experience, we knew three PVCs heralded problems down the road and should be treated. I am not certain what degree of change is important in $S\bar{v}O_2$. To go from 70% to 60% is of interest, but we do not have any documentation showing that that is of any clinical significance. As $S\bar{v}O_2$ moves into the 50% range, and certainly below 50%, I become much more concerned in terms of not meeting oxygen demands of the tissues. In terms of an absolute change of 5% or 10%, I usually look at the patient and investigate it; however, many times I will not do anything.

MCMICHAN: We also need to remember the degree of accuracy of the device itself. If you take a laboratory co-oximeter as the gold standard, the saturation provided by this bedside co-oximeter is in the region of $\pm 1\%$ to $\pm 2\%$. If you are going to interpret a value, you need to keep this in mind. Accuracy also depends on adequate calibration of the machine at the outset of your monitoring of the patient. If you draw back too hard on the distal lumen of any pulmonary artery (PA) catheter, you will artifically raise the saturation. Thus, you may well be setting your bedside co-oximeter at an incorrect level. This needs to be watched.

QUESTION: What was the explanation for the increase in the $S\bar{v}O_2$ in a patient with gastric hemorrhage? Why did it not behave like any other drop in cardiac output?

GORE: I think it probably falls along the same line as septic shock. It was our feeling that probably the acute drop in hemoglobin or hematocrit was compensated for by an attempt by the patient to improve the cardiac output. It goes back to the old days of warm shock and cold shock. I think the initial response may have been to try to increase cardiac output in whatever way possible, be it a sudden surge of catecholamines, adrenalin, or whatever. When the cardiac output goes up, the $S\bar{v}O_2$ goes up. If you follow these patients long enough, as in the septic patient, it does not stay up very long. After three or four hours it was back down in the 30% range, and she was dead 12 to 14 hours later.

ABERMAN: It must be that the increase in cardiac output outweighed any fall in hemoglobin. An acute GI hemorrhage will not change the hemoglobin dramatically, but it will lead to compensatory mechanisms via catecholamines. A possible explanation would be that the cardiac output outweighed the fall in hemoglobin.

QUESTION: Did you find it more difficult to pass the pulmonary artery catheter that had fiberoptics in it? Did you find it lasted as long as a typical pulmonary artery catheter we have today? What kinds of special problems did you have in making it work well in the patients?

ABERMAN: We have been using it now for about a year. For the first 6 months we did have problems with the catheter in terms of getting from the right ventricle to the pulmonary artery. We assumed it had to do with the catheter or some characteristics of the catheter. In the last 6 months we have had no problems. Of course, some people might say that is because we are more expert in putting it in, but I think there have been improvements in the catheters. Judging by my house officers at the present time, they are just as anxious to put in that catheter as any other brand of pulmonary artery catheter. I feel we are essentially just as successful with inserting that catheter as we are with a regular catheter. We have left the catheters in for as long as six days. How long I keep it in is the same as for any thermodilution catheter. I know the insert says something like 72 hours; but I know most of us leave it in as long as we feel we need it, and we take it out as early as we feel we do not need it.

GORE: Being cardiologists, we were trained in stiff catheterization of the right heart. We use stiff catheters in the cath lab or when we do pulmonary embolisms. We have found it makes absolutely no difference what type of flow-directed catheter we put in.

QUESTION: Is it hard to break the fiberoptics?

MCMICHAN: I have nurses who have broken them just by pulling on the catheter.

ABERMAN: The people who break catheters are house officers, not nurses.

MCMICHAN: I agree with you. I have looked at these catheters from when I received a first model from the company up until the current model. I have been able to show statistically, and this has been submitted now, that the first model was far more difficult to insert into the pulmonary artery than was the nonfiberoptic catheter. However, the current model is statistically the same as the nonfiberoptic catheter in terms of the number of attempts that my residents take to get it floated into a wedge position.

QUESTION: I am a thoracic surgeon. Do you know of any data where this type of monitoring is used in predicting events in the OR just before or immediately after surgery, particularly heart surgery?

STEVENS: Yes, we have been using it in "high-risk" patients for a while. I can assure you that there are major changes in $S\bar{v}O_2$ that occur before the anesthesiologist is able to pick up other parameters on conventional monitors. On several occasions we have asked the anesthesiologist to measure cardiac outputs because we had major falls in $S\bar{v}O_2$. He reluctantly did them, noted the marked drop in output, and sprang into action. I think it is a much earlier warning device in some instances than conventional monitoring.

MCMICHAN: From an anesthesiologist's point of view, I agree with all that Dr. Stevens has said. I have had relatively less experience with this catheter in the OR because I do not do cardiac anesthesia; I do general anesthesia. Nevertheless, there are increasing indications to use this catheter in the general surgical population with which I work. I do anesthesia for repair of abdominal aortic aneurysms, and it is very helpful in this area of major vascular surgery. Certainly, patients who come to my OR who need minimal anesthesia techniques because they are too sick to be given drugs have a smoother intrasurgical course if I have this monitoring. Also, my degree of stress is much less if I have an accurately working catheter in the OR.

ABERMAN: Dr. McMichan, would you agree with this comment? Although not all patients under anesthesia for major operations need to have PA catheters inserted, if there is a strong enough indication to insert a thermodilution catheter, there is certainly a case to be made for inserting a catheter that measures $S\bar{v}O_2$.

MCMICHAN: I would support that statement to the ultimate, and that also applies to my practice in the ICU. I now find, from a cost-benefit point of view, that if a fiberoptic catheter is in place, measurements of cardiac output and arterial blood gases (ABGs) and time required by technicians and nurses decrease. I am happy to say that my nurses can now spend more time with the patient instead of looking at numbers, and my technicians can do therapy treatments rather than spending a lot of time punching cardiac outputs and drawing blood for ABG analyses.

FAHEY: I have had no personal experience with surgical patients; however, there is an abstract by an anesthesiologist at the Cleveland Clinic who has used it intraoperatively. He found that surgical patients who had a drop in $S\bar{v}O_2$ to below 60% for longer than 15 minutes, with no other associated changes in the commonly measured variables, were the patients who had the stormiest intraoperative and postoperative courses in terms of days in the recovery room, hypotensive episodes, etc. $S\bar{v}O_2$ did appear to be an early indicator of trouble down the road in that one published series.

STEVENS: This is one of the few instruments with which you can have a 24-hour record of everything that has happened on a manageable piece of paper that is no more than 2 or 3 ft long. It is very rewarding to come in in the morning to make rounds and reconstruct everything deleterious that has happened to the patient. This data can be correlated with nurses' notes and a variety of other things that heretofore would have been completely unknown if the tracing had not been available.

QUESTION: All of this sounds almost too good to be true. I wonder if we are all going to go back home and get an instrument and start using it. I think it would probably be reasonable to do so. However, I do not think we should lose sight of whether or not this is or is not a penicillin. How do we ever evaluate whether or not it affects survival? Is that being systematically looked at?

ABERMAN: It is really that the technology has caught up to what has been known regarding physiology for a long time. I do not think any of us has said anything today that has not been said about $S\bar{v}O_2$ the last 30 or 40 years in the physiology literature. The difference is that we can measure it. We are not here to say that this is a major discovery that has been made in the last 2 years because it really is not.

A more difficult question to answer is this: Does it affect survival? I wish I knew whether the ICU itself affected survival, let alone a catheter. We know the ICU affects survival of drug overdose patients, for example. However, we really do not know the net effect of all ICU interventions. I think we should ask about the benefit ratio that affects survival. The major issue for me is whether or not to put in a PA line. We take a patient who is not on instruments, and we do a major intervention by putting in a PA line. We do a subclavian puncture with the attendant risks; we keep a line in with the real risk of sepsis. A major decision is made in any patient when you go from no monitoring to invasive monitoring. I do not feel that a major decision is made when you go from a thermodilution catheter to one that has a fiberoptic bundle. I do not see any additional risk to the patient. The real risk is to go from no monitoring to monitoring.

The financial issues today are real ones with diagnosis-related groups (DRGs) in the United States and similar concerns in Canada. You heard some people say that it may decrease costs because of ancillary benefits such as fewer measurements of blood gases and cardiac output.

FAHEY: There seems to be a small group of coronary bypass patients who have a prolonged metabolic acidosis that lasts three to five hours in the immediate postoperative period. Has anyone looked at mixed venous oxygen content in the immediate postoperative period? These patients seemed to have normal cardiac outputs and oxygen pressures (PO_2).

ABERMAN: Is it a lactic acidosis or a non-ionic gap hyperchloremic acidosis?

FAHEY: It is an ionic gap acidosis. There might be lactic acid that is washing out.

ABERMAN: Yes, there is a washout phenomenon.

GORE: I have seen it also, but we have not put this particular catheter in any of our bypass patients.

ABERMAN: For the first five or six hours you see lactate go up, not dramatically, not to ten, but from my experience from 1½ to three clear-cut elevations. Not really dramatic. I have never seen it in coronary bypass surgery.

GORE: You see it in valvular cases. I think it has to do with the length of the procedure more than how long the heart is cross-clamped.

QUESTION: Have any of you gentlemen noticed any thrombi due to the optical fibers? Associated with that, have you seen increased incidents of pulmonary emboli and baseline shifts due to attenuation of the signals because of encapsulation of the optical fibers?

FAHEY: There are some data that suggest that a noncalibrated catheter left in over a period of time will show a drift in accuracy. It was suggested that the drift was possibly due to clot formation. I do not think it has ever been proven that a clot was forming on the tip. We have found with daily calibration that there is no change in accuracy. It is just as accurate on Day 5 as it was on Day 1. Certainly, we have not seen any substantial changes that we could attribute to a pulmonary embolism or thrombus formation. I have seen reports of thrombi forming in up to 30% of pulmonary artery catheters. That has not been a clinical problem in our experience with this catheter or previous pulmonary artery catheters.

ABERMAN: Do not forget that the fiberoptics are not exposed to blood. The catheter is covered with the same material as other catheters. I do not think there is any reason fiberoptics per se will lead to increased thrombi.

FAHEY: These catheters are heparin coated or heparin treated. I have been using these catheters a long time, and I have found nothing on the catheters when I have pulled them out. The patients do not suddenly become hypoxic or develop chest pain. From the animal studies we are doing, it looks like the clot forms not only on the catheter but also on the wall of the heart. With time the clot endothelializes and disappears. I think we are going to find with more studies that it is not actually a thrombus on the catheter but that the thrombus is where the catheter comes in contact with the heart structures. With time the body's own thrombolytic mechanism will dissolve it.

MCMICHAN: We have just done such a study by taking all the hearts out of the patients who died in our institution during a 1-year period in whom a pulmonary artery catheter was in place. We looked for evidence of thrombi and mural damage in the right side of the heart and found it in about 40% of the patients.

Heparin-bonded or heparin-coated catheters have been forced upon us, whether or not we want them. I do not believe we need them. Perhaps we can show there is a role for heparin coating by repeating a study such as we have just done. We can see if there is a difference in mural or thrombotic lesions within the hearts of patients who die with a catheter in place. In fact, we are currently undertaking such a study.

QUESTION: Work presented at this convention concerning this particular question demonstrated that coating on a catheter made absolutely no difference in the rate of thrombus formation. Even heparinized saline flushing did not affect the number of thrombi around the catheters.

MCMICHAN: I agree with that entirely, and that has been my thought on this matter. We have never heparin coated all the central lines we have been putting in all these years. Why should we suddenly heparin coat these?

GORE: Just for the record, I disagree. I feel strongly that all catheters should be heparin coated.

MCMICHAN: There is no clinical evidence that says they need to be.

GORE: Dr. Hoar wrote in his letter to the Editor in the *New England Journal of Medicine* (305:993-995, 1981) about his findings in open-heart patients at the time of surgery. Ten out of ten catheters that were not treated with heparin had clots on them, while only one out of ten with heparin coating had a clot. This was a short time. I think heparin is something that may be good for 12 to 24 hours.

MCMICHAN: The clots in Hoar's patients did not cause any difficulty in the patients.

GORE: Yes, I agree.

QUESTION: Why is $S\bar{v}O_2$ superior to mixed venous oxygen tension in monitoring critically ill patients?

ABERMAN: I do not think anyone said that $S\bar{v}O_2$ is superior to mixed venous PO_2. Perhaps, if we had the technology to measure the mixed venous PO_2 continuously rather than the $S\bar{v}O_2$, we would have to address that issue. However, the only catheter around today measures $S\bar{v}O_2$. At the present time it is the only game in town.

$S\bar{v}O_2$ is determined by cardiac output, oxygen consumption, hemoglobin, and arterial saturation. If you tell me those four things, you have fixed $S\bar{v}O_2$. If you have changes in the position of the oxyhemoglobin dissociation curve caused by metabolic acidosis or anything else, you cannot get a change in $S\bar{v}O_2$ because it is fixed by the other four variables. Therefore, mixed venous PO_2 goes up. It is not changes in $S\bar{v}O_2$ that can mislead you when you have metabolic acidosis, but rather it is changes in mixed venous PO_2.

John Downs's experiment with dogs, in which he infused bicarbonate, showed that very effect. He infused bicarbonate and changed the position of the curve while keeping the other factors constant. The mixed venous PO_2 changed rather than the $S\bar{v}O_2$. A more fundamental physiological question is whether PO_2 on a tissue basis may be more important than saturation. It is PO_2 that is the pressure cascade. That is a different kind of question than a monitoring question.

STEVENS: What you say is true in the steady state. We are, however, not talking about a steady state in this situation. I am not sure which direction the various factors would go, but if you drop pH, you are going to drop both the arterial and the venous saturation. You are not going to change the arterial-venous oxygen saturation difference necessarily, which is a steady-state measurement. Unless you are sure the arterial stays 100% saturated, any change in arterial due to changes in the pH will be reflected in the venous.

ABERMAN: As a Canadian, I really admire at times like this the great American, Al Capone, who said, "It is easier to convince someone with a gun and a kind word than a kind word alone." I do not agree, but we will leave it at that.

ANSWERS TO PRETEST

1. b
2. a
3. c
4. a
5. d
6. d
7. d
8. a

CONTINUOUS MEASUREMENT OF BLOOD OXYGEN SATURATION IN THE HIGH RISK PATIENT

POSTTEST INSTRUCTIONS

The following questions are based on the entire monograph. Educational objectives are identified on page xiv. The purpose of this self-paced learning program is to increase your understanding of the principles and clinical applications of continuous $S\bar{v}O_2$ measurement in the high-risk patient.

There is only one correct answer to each test item. A score of 75% (22 correct answers) must be achieved to receive CE credit. Answers must be submitted on the answer form found on page 99 (you may make a copy of the answer form). Your test will be scored and returned to you along with your CE certificate. If you do not achieve a 75% passing score, you may retake the test. There is a charge of 25% of the enrollment fee if cancellation is required.

The answer sheet and CE enrollment information are found on page 99. For further information, contact:

Health Education International, Inc.
P.O. Box 28364
San Diego, CA 92128
(619) 451-0342

CONTINUOUS MEASUREMENT OF BLOOD OXYGEN SATURATION IN THE HIGH RISK PATIENT

POSTTEST

1. Major drawbacks in the early *in vivo* oximeters included all of the following *EXCEPT:*
   a. The stiffness and fragility of fiberoptic catheters
   b. The requirement for a two-point calibration of the system
   c. The need for large pieces of equipment to analyze the data
   d. The inability to compensate for periodic vessel wall artifact

2. The method used for *in vivo* measurement of mixed venous oxygen saturation involves:
   a. Counting oxygen molecules
   b. Analyzing light reflected by the blood cells
   c. Tagging oxyhemoglobin
   d. Comparing weight difference between hemoglobin and oxyhemoglobin

3. With the OXIMETRIX® Opticath® Oximetry System, carboxyhemoglobin is detected:
   a. As an almost nonabsorbing substance
   b. The same as oxyhemoglobin
   c. As an opaque substance
   d. Only if present in large amounts

4. The optical module portion of the OXIMETRIX Opticath Oximetry System is the:
   a. Source of calibration
   b. Optical and electrical interface
   c. Microprocessor
   d. Most frequently broken portion

5. The OXIMETRIX Processor provides all of the following *EXCEPT:*
   a. Continuous chart recording
   b. Digital display of oxygen saturation
   c. Light intensity display to demonstrate accuracy
   d. Analysis of waveform characteristics

6. The standardization technique used in the OXIMETRIX Opticath Oximetry System allows calibration against:
   a. Normal blood samples
   b. An absolute color standard
   c. Atmospheric light waves
   d. Atmospheric pressure

7. As compared to the arterial system, in the venous system small changes in PO_2 will result in:
   a. Large changes in venous O_2 saturation
   b. Small changes in arterial O_2 saturation
   c. Small changes in venous O_2 saturation
   d. No changes in O_2 saturation

8. Oxygen content is:
   a. Primarily a product of dissolved oxygen
   b. Primarily a product of saturated oxygen
   c. Equally a product of dissolved and saturated oxygen
   d. A product of cardiac output and dissolved oxygen

9. Oxygen consumption can be expressed as:
   a. Cardiac output × hemoglobin × 13.8 × A-V saturation difference
   b. Cardiac output × hemoglobin × 1.38 × arterial saturation
   c. 13.8 × venous saturation × cardiac output
   d. Hemoglobin × A-V saturation difference

10. A decrease in the value for hemoglobin will have which of the following effects on the oxygen consumption formula if all else remains unchanged?
   a. No change
   b. Decrease in value
   c. Increase in value
   d. Cannot be determined

11. To prevent lactic acidosis it is important that:
   a. O_2 consumption exceed O_2 demand
   b. O_2 demand exceed O_2 consumption
   c. O_2 consumption equal O_2 demand
   d. None of the above

12. Compensatory mechanisms to maintain O_2 consumption at an acceptable value include:
   a. Decrease in cardiac output
   b. Increase in $S\bar{v}O_2$
   c. Increase in cardiac output
   d. Increase in hemoglobin

13. The greatest threat to the O_2 consumption formula is a:
   a. Decrease in cardiac output
   b. Decrease in arterial O_2 saturation
   c. Increase in venous O_2 saturation
   d. Decrease in hemoglobin

14. Changes in venous oxygen content in the cardiac patient can be assumed to represent changes in:
   a. Myocardial oxygenation
   b. Systemic vascular resistance
   c. Preload
   d. Cardiac output

15. Oxygen saturations of 82% in the right atrium, 74% in the right ventricle, and 68% in the pulmonary artery would be most characteristic of:
   a. Ventricular septal defect
   b. Right ventricular failure
   c. Atrial septal defect
   d. Normal intracardiac saturations

16. During insertion of the OXIMETRIX catheter, O_2 saturations should be recorded in each chamber as a diagnostic run. Normal results would be:
   a. Very little change in values
   b. Atrial $S\bar{v}O_2$ greater than ventricular $S\bar{v}O_2$
   c. PA $S\bar{v}O_2$ dramatically higher than ventricular $S\bar{v}O_2$
   d. Steady reduction in values

17. The diagnostic run can be useful in diagnosing:
   a. Coronary artery disease
   b. Septal defects
   c. Ventricular hypertrophy
   d. Pulmonary hypertension

18. With continuous monitoring of $S\bar{v}O_2$, a deleterious event in the patient may be indicated by:
   a. A dramatic increase in the saturation value
   b. A dramatic decrease in the saturation value
   c. Either a dramatic increase or decrease in the saturation value
   d. A dramatic increase in the intensity bars

19. Continuous $S\bar{v}O_2$ monitoring in the coronary care unit may result in:
   a. Need for additional personnel
   b. Prolonged ICU stay
   c. Decreased costs
   d. Increased blood sampling

20. $S\bar{v}O_2$ monitoring can be useful in:
   a. Weaning patients from intra-aortic balloon counterpulsation
   b. Determining prognosis
   c. Weaning patients from mechanical ventilation
   d. All of the above

21. A progressive decrease in $S\bar{v}O_2$ values usually antedates:
   a. Serious hemodynamic deterioration
   b. Misplacement of the OXIMETRIX catheter
   c. Deterioration of arterial PCO_2
   d. Cardiac dysrhythmias

22. In evaluating $S\bar{v}O_2$ levels, it is important to remember that the two major determinants of $S\bar{v}O_2$ are:
   a. Oxygen consumption and cardiac output
   b. Arterial O_2 content and cardiac output response to tissue O_2 demand
   c. Arterial saturation and oxygen consumption
   d. Pulmonary vascular resistance and cardiac output

23. Monitoring during coughing episodes in the patient with respiratory failure has shown:
  a. Mild increases in O_2 consumption
  b. Dramatic increases in cardiac output
  c. Dramatic decreases in arterial O_2 saturation
  d. Dramatic decreases in $S\bar{v}O_2$ levels

24. Clinical experience with $S\bar{v}O_2$ monitoring has demonstrated that during endotracheal suctioning:
  a. $S\bar{v}O_2$ and arterial O_2 levels decrease the same amount
  b. $S\bar{v}O_2$ levels remain constant while arterial O_2 levels decrease
  c. $S\bar{v}O_2$ levels decrease much more than arterial O_2 levels
  d. $S\bar{v}O_2$ levels actually increase while arterial O_2 levels decrease

25. Continuous $S\bar{v}O_2$ monitoring has been used as an indication of the effects of various modes of ventilatory assistance on:
  a. The oxygen cost of breathing
  b. The degree of barotrauma incurred
  c. Pulmonary vascular resistance
  d. Respiratory drive

26. The level of PEEP at which cardiopulmonary function is compromised rather than enhanced can be determined most readily by observing for:
  a. An increase in heart rate
  b. An $S\bar{v}O_2$ value of 90%
  c. A decrease in $S\bar{v}O_2$
  d. A decrease in blood pressure

27. Monitoring of $S\bar{v}O_2$ provides feedback of changes occurring in:
  a. Cardiopulmonary function or tissue oxygen consumption
  b. Pulmonary vasculature or cardiac function
  c. Arterial saturation or tissue oxygen consumption
  d. Metabolic rate or pulmonary function

28. In any form of hemodynamic deterioration, which value will most quickly demonstrate the event?
  a. Mean arterial pressure
  b. Cardiac output
  c. $S\bar{v}O_2$
  d. Heart rate

29. A dramatic increase in $S\bar{v}O_2$ values may indicate:
   a. Catacholamine-induced increase in cardiac output
   b. Decrease in tissue oxygen consumption
   c. Increase in tissue oxygen supply
   d. Dramatic decrease in cardiac output

30. An occult bleeding episode in a high-risk patient may be demonstrated by:
   a. An increase in $S\bar{v}O_2$ due to a compensatory increase in cardiac output
   b. A decrease in $S\bar{v}O_2$ due to decreased hemoglobin
   c. An increase in $S\bar{v}O_2$ due to decreased hemoglobin with increased saturation
   d. A decrease in the number of intensity bars, indicating decreased blood flow

ANSWER SHEET AND ENROLLMENT FORM

INSTRUCTIONS:

- Use only this form to submit your answers for CE Credit. (You may make a copy of this page.)
- Select one answer for each question.
- Mark your answers clearly by placing an "X" in the box next to the correct answer.

  Example: ☐ a
  ☒ b
  ☐ c
  ☐ d

- Passing score is 75% (22 correct answers).
- To enroll for CE, complete the form provided below and submit with your answers.
- For your convenience, Answer Sheet/Enrollment Form may be detached, folded, and mailed. (Address is preprinted on back.)

1. ☐ a ☐ b ☐ c ☐ d	**2.** ☐ a ☐ b ☐ c ☐ d	**3.** ☐ a ☐ b ☐ c ☐ d	**4.** ☐ a ☐ b ☐ c ☐ d	**5.** ☐ a ☐ b ☐ c ☐ d	**6.** ☐ a ☐ b ☐ c ☐ d	**7.** ☐ a ☐ b ☐ c ☐ d	**8.** ☐ a ☐ b ☐ c ☐ d	**9.** ☐ a ☐ b ☐ c ☐ d	**10.** ☐ a ☐ b ☐ c ☐ d
11. ☐ a ☐ b ☐ c ☐ d	**12.** ☐ a ☐ b ☐ c ☐ d	**13.** ☐ a ☐ b ☐ c ☐ d	**14.** ☐ a ☐ b ☐ c ☐ d	**15.** ☐ a ☐ b ☐ c ☐ d	**16.** ☐ a ☐ b ☐ c ☐ d	**17.** ☐ a ☐ b ☐ c ☐ d	**18.** ☐ a ☐ b ☐ c ☐ d	**19.** ☐ a ☐ b ☐ c ☐ d	**20.** ☐ a ☐ b ☐ c ☐ d
21. ☐ a ☐ b ☐ c ☐ d	**22.** ☐ a ☐ b ☐ c ☐ d	**23.** ☐ a ☐ b ☐ c ☐ d	**24.** ☐ a ☐ b ☐ c ☐ d	**25.** ☐ a ☐ b ☐ c ☐ d	**26.** ☐ a ☐ b ☐ c ☐ d	**27.** ☐ a ☐ b ☐ c ☐ d	**28.** ☐ a ☐ b ☐ c ☐ d	**29.** ☐ a ☐ b ☐ c ☐ d	**30.** ☐ a ☐ b ☐ c ☐ d

ENROLLMENT INFORMATION

Please enroll me in the CE program: CONTINUOUS MEASUREMENT OF BLOOD OXYGEN SATURATION IN THE HIGH RISK PATIENT

Fee $18.00 (U.S. Dollars) CE Credit Hours: 3

Add $2.00 for addresses outside the continental United States and in foreign countries.

Name ______________________ State of Licensure ____________
(Please print clearly)

Social Security No. ______-______-______ and License No. ____________

Address ______________________

City ______________________ State ____________ Zip ____________

Specialty Area ______________________

☐ My check (or money order) payable to Health Education International, Inc., is enclosed.

☐ Bill my MasterCard/Visa Number (circle one):

Card No. ______________________ Expires ____________

Signature ______________________

☐ I have enclosed an additional $21.00 for Air Express delivery.

☐ I have enclosed an additional $7.00 for rush delivery.

OX/1/1/85

(Staple Here)

(Fold Here)

Place
Stamp
Here

Health Education International, Inc.
P.O. Box 28364
San Diego, CA 92128